SOUL STRENGTH

PETER N. NIELSEN

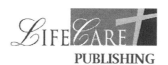
LifeCare
PUBLISHING

Principles of Hope website: http://principlesofhope.com/

Principles of Hope facebook page:
https://www.facebook.com/pages/Principles-of-Hope/266504550054343

LifeCare Publishing is a branch of
LifeCare Christian Center
A non-profit faith-based ministry
www.LifeCareChristianCenter.org
info.lifecarecc@gmail.com
Westland, MI USA

Mission Statement
LifeCare Christian Center exists to partner with individuals, churches and the community in promoting spiritual, emotional, physical and relational wholeness, by providing quality, affordable care, education and training services from a Christian perspective.

ISBN-13: 978-0692023853 (LifeCare Publishing)

ISBN-10: 0692023852

To my two daughters, Erika and Dana

who have truly given me the reasons to believe again.
After having no direction on how to be a father, they brought me closer
to the Lord, wanting to search for answers on His love; and through that,
the healing process began. And not only was I more capable of
reflecting Jesus' love to my daughters, but it gave me the hope to spread
the good news to the world.
So every day that I get up, I look at my two daughters and see God's
love. I will be forever grateful for those two amazing gifts that He has
given me that are more important than any title, any TV show, any book
or any fortune.

ACKNOWLEDGMENTS

First and foremost, Christ, my Lord and Savior. Thank You for loving me, for guiding me, for giving me Your mercy and grace and uncommon favor, after I finally allowed You in my life. I want to thank you for teaching me Your love so I can reflect it to others.

My kids: Dana and Erika, for also teaching me unconditional love and giving me the reasons to get up every morning to truly finish strong no matter how I was programmed when I was born. You rewired me with God's love to truly understand grace, hope, peace, light and joy. I forever thank you.

Pastor Paul. After not having a good father role model, God knew what I needed and when. He brought you into my life over 30 years ago as a beacon of light who became my spiritual dad. I am forever thankful for you adjusting my moral compass.

Asaad. Thank you for allowing the Lord to be a bridge in connecting so many dots, and for your endless love.

For Mike and Lillian Smith, thank you for your patience, for your hearts, for bringing my words to life through this book, *Soul Strength*. Forever grateful for our friendship.

David Rutz. Thank you for being obedient to God in a Starbucks coffee shop and coming up to me and introducing yourself. It was a life changer.

Mark Jarvis and Jay Shafer. Thank you for allowing me to be a part of something so big. Thank you for being obedient in helping broaden the platform of the ministry of Principles of Hope.

Kelly Hawkins. Thank you for putting this book in production and on paper. Your patience and endless hours on editing and publishing will be forever remembered.

Pastor Brad Powell. Thank you for your leadership, for your spiritual guidance and for always telling it like it is, never bending His Word, never watering down a message and always truly spreading the gospel.

CONTENTS

FOREWORD

On a Sunday morning in 1987, Peter Nielsen received Christ into his life at the church where I was the pastor. For twenty-six years our paths were separated. We were divinely reunited in August 2011. Now, as spiritual father and son, we have the exciting privilege of ministering together, proclaiming God's "Soul Strength" for broken lives in our hopelessly broken world. That's why Peter has published his private and personal thoughts about God's grace and love to his own soul.

It is often said that dynamite comes in small packages. This book fulfills that adage. It will prove to be a living explosion of relevant and practical strength and encouragement from the Source of all wisdom, Jesus Christ, as it flows into your soul and spirit. Peter's deeply personal and practical commitment to, and his undeniable love for God, will challenge you to walk the walk with him.

When you know the story of God's love in his life, you will understand more fully why Peter often says his greatest desire is to finish his race strong for the sake of Christ. His passionate prayer is to live to see thousands of people, like you and me, experience the healing, hope and wholeness of spirit, soul and body, that he received through being committed to Christ.

Peter has become known as the Health, Wholeness, and Fitness expert on his nationally syndicated TV and Radio shows, airing on major networks across America. After adding a degree in Nutrition, Peter experienced an ever increasing audience, watching and listening to "Peter's Principles." This resulted in changed lives, because of his challenge to capture the principles of better nutrition, better health, better fitness and new hope.

In 2001, God spoke to him, saying, "Peter, do you love and trust Me enough to boldly use the national platforms I have given you, to declare My Name on your shows?" Since then he speaks clearly, about the power of Jesus Christ to bring new hope for living in Health, Wholeness, and Fitness in your spirit, soul and body. Peter calls it, "Soul Strength" because God says He desires that "...we will be in health and prosper, as our soul prospers." (3 John 2)

The ministry of Peter's new venture, "Soul Strength", began with that challenge. He enjoys telling anyone who will listen, that hope is the confident expectation that Almighty God will keep His promises. He defines hope as "Having Optimum Positive Emotions about those situations in your life that seem to be impossible." It requires trusting the living God for the hope you need to "give Him one more day" to change your life, just as Peter experienced nearly thirty years ago!

Welcome to "Soul Strength", inspiringly proclaimed by Peter Nielsen!

Paul Bersche

ABOUT THE AUTHOR

Peter N. Nielsen

Life has not always been a mountain top experience for Peter. Having grown up with emotional and physical scars from an abusive father and the tough streets of Brooklyn, he had yet to face his toughest opponent. At age 15, Peter was diagnosed with an incurable disease called Crohn's. After a major surgery and many consultations with doctors, the word *hope* was becoming a distant memory, and life looked very bleak for this very sick teenager. No one, including the doctors, seemed to know how to help.

Two dark years later, just seconds before Peter was to take his own life, he heard God's unmistakable loving voice say, "Give me one more day, Peter." Peter accepted that challenge, and he began a life-long journey to spiritual, physical, and emotional wholeness and living out soul strength. This amazing journey of almost 30 years has included over 50 body building titles. Peter is also known as the health, wholeness, and fitness expert on nationally syndicated TV and radio shows airing on major networks. He has been a much sought after trainer for thousands who have relied on his whole person tailor-made approach to wellness.

On March 7, 2001, the Crohn's disease reared its ugly head and again challenged Peter's life. At 2:14 AM his heart stopped beating for 43 seconds. During the miraculous recovery that followed, God once again spoke a clear message into the depths of Peter's heart. "Peter, do you love and trust me enough to boldly use your national platform to declare My name on your shows?" As a result, Peter now speaks passionately and without reserve about the true and lasting hope that is found only in Jesus Christ. That surrender has led to his ministry, Principles of Hope, which is now reaching people across the world.

God continues to spread the truth through Peter that we can have the confident expectation that God will keep His promises, and that His hope never disappoints. Jesus is the "living hope" you can anchor your life upon. Give Him "one more day" so that He can change your life in a radical way just as Peter experienced almost 30 years ago.

INTRODUCTION

"Show me a person who found their passion, and I'll show you a person
living a purposeful life."
– P. N. N.

"I have said these things to you, that in me you may have peace. In the
world you will have tribulation. But take heart; I have overcome the
world."
– John 16:33, ESV

Welcome friends!

Does controlled chaos describe your everyday life? Have the deep hurts of your past paralyzed your ability to forgive? Has your addiction tried to give you one last knockout punch to ensure you never again try another recovery? Or is it that your tank is just on empty from auto-pilot living and life without purpose?

This amazing journey we're on dishes out unexpected twists and turns that jump out at us like thieves in the night, robbing us of every last ounce of joy and strength we possess.

Dark days of turmoil and regret loom over us like ominous storm clouds that never give way to the sun. Minor setbacks that were once easy to maneuver can become mountains that all too often are impossible to scale. Let's face it, life can go from a whisper to a roar in a New York second leaving us reeling and muttering, or at times screaming at the top of our lungs, "I can't do this anymore!"

"There is an answer to your problem,

and there is freedom from the bondage!"

If what I'm describing here is what your life looks like right now, be of good cheer. Believe it or not, it is here that there is hope and strength; here, where God's very voice cries out to you. It says, "There *is* an answer to your problem, and there *is* freedom from the bondage!" There *is* a peace in the midst of this raging storm! You are worth it! God says in His Word, there *will* be trials and temptations, struggles and setbacks, but He has the answer; in fact, He *is* the answer! There is something your Creator has placed in the deepest core of your being that, honestly, not many *ever* tap into, but it contains the very life you were meant to live! I call it Soul Strength! Imagine never having to stay in the constant season of sorrow or be taken by temptation. God wants you to be unleashed from the beast of burden that continues to hold you captive. This is not pie in the sky thinking or the good life every late night infomercial offers, and it's not the false hope sold on every corner packaged in self-help books or Hollywood propaganda. Those, at best, are temporary emotional highs that lead you on a short trip to disappointment, and at worst, will leave you with deep regret, picking up pieces of one bad decision after another. In short, they don't work!

Let me be clear about this book. This book is not a method or another in a long line of "how to" manuals. It's about the voice and power of the living God, your Creator, the One who knit you together in your mother's womb. He sees, He understands, He comforts, He heals! If you're not a believer, I welcome you to this journey with open arms, and I have a grateful heart that you're here! You are like a deep mine where there are priceless, precious gems, but to find them you must dig deep and have patience. When they are finally found, you will be able to enjoy true riches that have eternal value and fill you with joy beyond compare! My prayer is that this book will provoke your spirit, press your buttons, push you beyond your limits, and propel your life from the sidelines to the frontlines.

One last thing before we begin our sojourn from the inside out: I believe in being completely honest, so I will tell you the truth. I stole much of this book, even the very idea from another author. His name is Jesus, the Author of life, the Author of soul strength! The heartbeat of my life is to lead others to know Him and to experience the abundant life He offers. Getting to know Him has turned my tragedy into triumph and my adversity into advantage.

So…let's begin, and get better together!

– Peter

CHAPTER 1

SOUL STRENGTH

"Dear friend, I pray that you are doing well in every way and that you are
healthy, just as your soul is healthy."
– 3 John 1:2, ISV

As many of you know, I am all about physical training, and that is immensely important. I pray you never forget that truth. Physical training has a direct connection to your mind, emotions, and your spirit. There is, however, training that we so often neglect, or really may not even know about, that affects every aspect of our lives. Life decisions, relationships, career, and yes, even health are deeply affected by it on every level.

It is the training of the spirit.

Being spiritually fit is what Soul Strength is all about. God's, not Peter's, principles will build and strengthen the very core of who you are and enable you to become what you were designed to be. Whether you know it or not, you have an enemy who wants to destroy you from the inside out, and sometimes from the outside in. If you have a weak spiritual foundation, your chances of being devoured are very likely. We've all seen mansions, marriages, and minds crumbled by a lack of spiritual wisdom and discernment. Look at the long trail of carnage left behind in the political, sports, and entertainment worlds. People who appear to have it all together, and are seen almost as gods in this world, are suddenly the joke of the tabloids and the disgrace of their families. How different would it be if Tiger Woods or Bill Clinton had trained their spirit and understood soul strength? Many legacies have been destroyed by those who chose immediate gratification over godly wisdom.

Many times we limp and stagger around the same block 480 times and can't figure out why. The reason is that we don't hear God's directive and loving voice. Like no other time in history has our mind been under siege by the voice of the enemy. Our eyes and ears are inundated with messages that war against truth and honesty. We are a society with a deadly disease called "us." We leave no margin and are multitasking ourselves to a frazzle. We attempt to text ourselves to deeper relationships and are deathly afraid of being alone and in silence.

In the television business there is a term we use called Nat sound, or natural sound. It's the vague sounds you hear but can't make out when someone is talking behind closed doors, or like a radio playing off in the distance. You know there is sound, but can't understand what is being said. When we busy ourselves with us, to do's, and the world's agenda, the very voice of God our Creator, the One who can tell you the very next step you need to take, and who can warn you of coming danger, becomes the Nat sound in your life. This is why we are continually tripping over ourselves. If we're continually looking

Are you living a purposeful life?

Do you feel like an actor in a play who doesn't know the script?

over a burdened shoulder that's carrying a tall stack of worry-weights and a ton of to-do's, with no sign of peace, this should be a bright warning or check engine light in our lives that we need soul strength.

God has given us an amazing, powerful, and sometimes dangerous gift called free choice. We can accept Him and learn to listen to His voice or reject Him and live life randomly, often with tragic consequences. It's as simple as that. I've seen many living examples of both: those who follow God's direction in their choices and those who reject His direction and follow their own ways. My plea and prayer for you is that you choose to listen to His voice and follow Him in the choices you make.

Asking God into every part of your life can light a fire in your heart and spirit that will change the course of your existence now and forever. The foundation you need burned into your DNA is one that is embodied and endorsed by His Word, the Bible. As I said earlier, God tells us there will be times of trial, heartache, and temptation. The game changer of life is how we respond to them. The proper response can only be found in the soul strength that He gives when we know Him and the power of His Word. The script of your life can be changed dramatically and the rest of the chapters end victoriously with soul strength.

Let me ask you a couple questions, whether you're a believer or not. Are you living a purposeful life? Do you feel like an actor in a play who doesn't know the script? The core of soul strength is the very voice of God who can tell you what your role is, how to play it, how to deal with the other actors in it, and how to make the last scene the best scene that includes an eternal curtain call! Without soul strength nothing is too small to take you down, and with it, nothing is too big that can't be taken down. It starts simply by asking God to reveal His true self to you, grabbing onto the hope that He has already burned into your soul, and trusting Him to be your provider for your life. He is not waiting with a hammer of judgment, but with

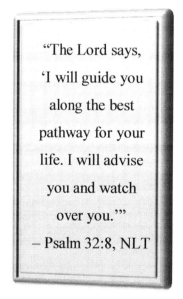

"The Lord says, 'I will guide you along the best pathway for your life. I will advise you and watch over you.'"
– Psalm 32:8, NLT

the tender hands of a loving Father who wants you to have His heart and mind on every matter.

You hold this book in your hand for a reason. God has been pursuing you all of your life with wild abandon. He has been in the fire with you. He has shared your grief and sufferings. In fact, if you are alive and reading this book, make no mistake about it—He has brought you through *every* trial, every heartache, and every situation you've ever faced. He has a very detailed and amazing plan for you right now. This is the day the Lord has made, and with soul strength you can rejoice in it and live with the power of His spirit guiding you along each and every step of your journey.

"The Lord says, 'I will guide you along the best pathway for your life. I will advise you and watch over you.'" – Psalm 32:8, NLT

H.O.P.E.

Having Optimum Positive Emotions
– P.N.N.

Hope to me is <u>H</u>aving <u>O</u>ptimum <u>P</u>ositive <u>E</u>motions about something that seems nearly impossible. Hope will see the invisible, feel the intangible, and if you allow it to, will accomplish the impossible. I'm speaking here of God's promise of hope that He gives everyone through His Son and His Word.

Hope: Problem or Promise?

Hope becomes a problem when the object of it cannot deliver what it promised. Here are some of the usual suspects our enemy and the world use as tempting lures to hook us into false hope: fame, alcohol, drugs, and gambling try with futility to fill a spiritual hole with a fleshly desire. I call these Hollywood Hopes. They're just actors making you feel good for a short time.

When you put your hope in these false gods, they disappoint and deceive you. Eventually your mind says to you, "See, I told you there was no such thing. Hope is just an overused word that eventually brings disappointment."

If we allow ourselves to, we can fall into the deepest pit of this complete lie just as German philosopher Friedrich Nietzsche did when he said, "Hope in reality is the worst of all evils because it prolongs the torments of man." He believed hope just prolonged people's torment.

Hope can also become a problem when we put it in feelings. Our feelings can take us on a bumpy ride or a smooth glide at any given time. They are a notoriously false barometer of whether hope is real or not. Feelings should be passengers, not drivers. When you are feeling something, find out what caused the feeling to occur and why.

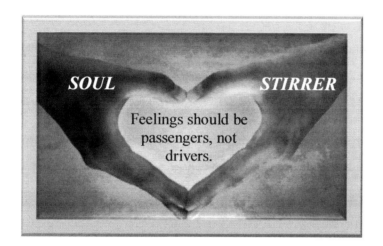

SOUL STIRRER

Feelings should be passengers, not drivers.

Hope as a Promise

Real hope has to have something immovable to hang onto.

When I started seeing hope as a promise from God Himself, it took on new life and was burned into my DNA. I started to believe and dig into the truth of God's Word. I stopped gambling my hope on the created, and I invested it in the Creator. Romans 15:13, NLT says, "I pray the God, the source of hope, will fill you completely with joy and peace because you trust in him. Then you will overflow with confident hope through the power of the Holy Spirit."

STRENGTH BUILDERS

1. What is your current definition of hope?

2. Does hope seem to be a problem or promise for you? And what exactly does that mean as you make it personal?

3. What are some things you have placed your hope in that didn't deliver what they promised?

How We Lose Our Hope

There is a multitude of things that can build what appears to be a strong case against hope in our lives. Here are three that really resonate with many people.

1. Circumstances

The range of circumstances in life you and I face is far and wide. You may be in the dark pit of devastation and shock over the loss of a loved one. Perhaps you're dealing with stress, confusion and anger as the result of an unforeseen job or financial loss, or a broken heart because a relationship has ended. Unfortunately, all of these scenarios paint a picture similar to my life's past, and possibly yours too.

2. Abuse

Many of us are all too aware of long seasons of pain and shame from abuse that could range from sexual to emotional and spiritual abuse. The scars I bore were deep and lasting. I often hid the pain, shame and unforgiveness because it seemed like the only thing I could do, but in reality, it held me captive as a slave to bitterness, and ultimately to hopelessness. Hiding pain, as well as other things such as anger and unforgiveness, is like burying something alive. Over time it will eventually fight its way to the surface.

3. Our past

Whether past actions that we're ashamed of or dreams that once had a place deep in our heart that have now somehow vanished, our past has a way of trying to hold us back from the hope of future possibilities. Often I tried, by my own power, to change my behavior, but it was short lived. You can't act your way out of brokenness; you must be healed to find hope.

STRENGTH BUILDERS

1. Of these three, circumstances, abuse, and your past, which have robbed you of hope and how?

One common denominator of failing in life is losing hope. The effects of losing it can be deeply destructive from the inside out. I can't emphasize this enough. Having found soul strength has stopped my past circumstances of abuse from calling hope a liar.

The hope that God gives may at times be tested, but it can always be trusted. His spirit helps us endure and His promises are true and faithful. I am living proof!

2. If your experience has been like mine, write about a time when hope was stirred in you and helped you go on. If not, what else keeps you from experiencing hope once again or being stirred?

> "And this hope will not lead to disappointment. For we know how dearly God loves us, because he has given us the Holy Spirit to fill our hearts with his love. When we were utterly helpless, Christ came at just the right time and died for us sinners."
> – Romans 5:5-6, NLT

_____

_____

_____

_____

_____

_____

_____

_____

_____

_____

_____

_____

_____

_____

_____

_____

_____

_____

_____

_____

My Living Hope Story

I would like to take you a little deeper into my journey to soul strength. It was at one of the darkest points in my life where hope was lost and ultimately restored. After being diagnosed with Crohn's disease at age fourteen, I was devastated. I left the hospital at a frail 86 pounds and came home to parents who had let the fear of my diagnosis turn into anger and blaming each other and our family history. I watched my dad become a raging and violent alcoholic who eventually tried to kill my mother. I remember that day as if it were yesterday. As I witnessed my mother turning blue from my father wrapping a telephone cord around her neck, I made a choice to go against my earthly father to save her life. She got away, but my father's rage continued and left me with six stitches above my eye and a collar bone broken in three places.

These tragic events coupled with the Crohn's diagnosis robbed me of any existing hope I was hanging onto. I felt I was left with one choice, to exit this hopeless world by taking my own life. On a bitter cold January night at 2am, as I made what I envisioned

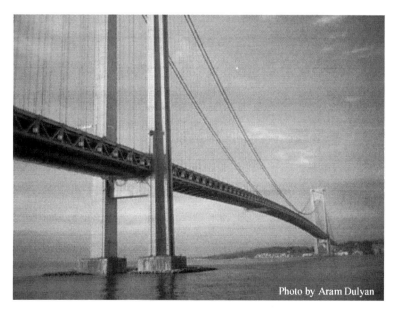

Photo by Aram Dulyan

would be my final trek to Brooklyn's Verrazano Bridge, I watched every last shred of hope vanish from my heart, and along with that, my will to live. After crying to the point that my eyes had almost swelled shut, I gave up and had lost all reason to go on.

My home was not a safe place, and my matrix of trust had been shattered. I knew no boundaries, and to me, hope *was* just a word that ended in disappointment. I didn't believe or want anything to do with God. But somehow that night I managed to shout at the heavens, "If You're there and You're real, God, I need You to get me out of here! I need Your help now!"

As I tearfully looked down at the razorblade which I had stolen from my dad's shaving kit (the tool which was to be the final fix to all my problems), I heard the voice of the promise keeper, the voice of God my Creator saying, "Give Me one more chance; give Me one more day." For

> *"Give Me one more chance;*
>
> *give Me one more day."*

a second I heard my own voice say I was a coward for not following through, but then the very voice of my Creator stopped me in my tracks and from allowing myself any more time to change my mind. I heaved the razorblade into the Hudson River. As I watched it skip across the water and then quickly disappear out of sight, I felt His undeniable presence and love sweep over me. It was then that I had my first real understanding of hope. I didn't fully realize it until years later, but God was standing right there with me, whispering *His* hope and soul strength to my spirit. By His grace, mercy and relentless pursuit of me, I stand here today with a testimony of real and proven hope!

No matter where you are, God says it's never too late to start again! He has already written your testimony. He's just asking you to trust Him to reveal it to you.

STRENGTH BUILDERS

1. How have you let past or present circumstances have control over your hope for the future?

2. Whose voice are you listening to as it relates to your hope for the future?

3. As you read Proverbs 3:5-6 on this page, reflect and write on times you have relied on your own understanding. What were the results?

> "Trust in the lord with all your heart; do not depend on your own understanding. Seek his will in all you do and he will show you which path to take."
> – Proverbs 3:5-6, NLT

_____

_____

_____

_____

_____

_____

_____

_____

_____

You may be in the darkest season of your life, but remember it's always darkest right before the dawn.

4. Write out a commitment statement to persevere through the process of finding hope and soul strength.

_____

_____

_____

_____

_____

_____

_____

_____

The Mind Connection

Once you really believe it's over, it's over!

Our mind is the fortress that is always under attack. What we fill our mind with, combined with our beliefs, is the recipe for either success or failure. It begins and ends in the mind!

If you're filling your mind with negative thoughts, ungodly music, and the media, they will win the war and steal your hope. You've heard the saying, "garbage in garbage out." If your mind is being filled with the garbage of the world, it can stay in for many years and will gain power over you until you push it out by the renewing of your mind through God's Word. The book of Romans chapter 12 verse 2 says, "Do not conform to the pattern of this world, but be transformed by the renewing of your mind. Then you will be able to test and approve what God's will is—his good, pleasing and perfect will." The product of this is soul strength.

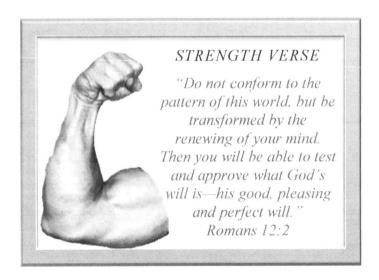

STRENGTH VERSE

"Do not conform to the pattern of this world, but be transformed by the renewing of your mind. Then you will be able to test and approve what God's will is—his good, pleasing and perfect will."
Romans 12:2

STRENGTH BUILDERS

1. What are the sources of input that need to be evaluated in your life that are filling your mind?

2. Are you being programmed for failure or success by what you're allowing to enter your mind?

3. What are the positive resources?

4. What are the negative resources?

Hope will always keep us moving forward—it looks to the future with an assurance that God will intercede. His interceding comes through relationship with Him.

He wants you to believe! He wants to connect with you. Remember that voice I told you about? It's Him calling out: "Give Me one more day; I am what you have been looking for all along!"

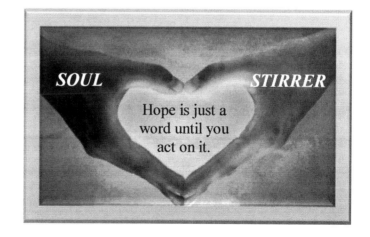

SOUL STIRRER

Hope is just a word until you act on it.

Restoring Hope

Restoring hope is a process and takes patience and time, but it is very much worth the effort!

There is a very powerful song with profound words called "A Thousand Steps" from the band New Song. It goes like this:

> *If there were a thousand steps between you and God*
> *and you could see no way across the great divide,*
> *just take one step towards His loving arms*
> *and He'll take nine hundred and ninety nine.*

Friends, it just takes one simple step to start restoring hope in your life. You must begin by believing there is hope for you and your life. There is something locked up deep within you desperately wanting to believe. Hope is the key to set it free.

Getting out of your own way is essential to hope. So many times we want full control over all of life. We can never change what happened in the past, but we can embrace today and the hope it brings. If you are alive today you can have hope!

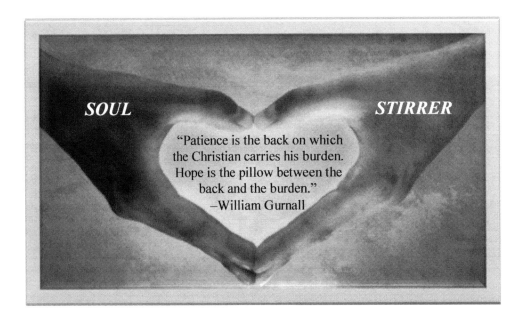

SOUL   STIRRER

"Patience is the back on which
the Christian carries his burden.
Hope is the pillow between the
back and the burden."
–William Gurnall

STRENGTH BUILDERS

I want you to take a minute and interview yourself. Dig deep and ask some questions of the heart.

1. Is there anything that could potentially be causing you to fear the future and fear taking the risk to hope again? If so, what is it?

   > "The Lord answered, 'If you had faith even as small as a mustard seed, you could say to this mulberry tree, "May you be uprooted and thrown into the sea," and it would obey you!'"
   > – Luke 17:6, NLT

2. Is there any other "wall" that is preventing you from moving forward and moving toward hope? Take some time to listen and reflect. What are you sensing God is saying to you?

"You can live weeks without food, days without water, minutes without the air you breathe, but without hope, you're finished in seconds. You're done.
– P.N.N.

Many people say to me they just don't believe. They just don't have hope. In those times, it encourages me and prompts me to share my testimony again and again because that's exactly where I was! When you don't believe, it's just you against you. It's a losing game. Trust me; a little faith can go a long way.

Often times hope comes in time—through a process. Hope gains power in patience, and loses power through pride.

I am reminded of the poem and picture called "Footprints in the Sand" (see below).

FOOTPRINTS IN THE SAND

One night a man had a dream.

He dreamed he was walking along the beach with the Lord. Across the sky flashed scenes from his life.

For each scene, he noticed two sets of footprints in the sand: one belonging to him, and the other to the Lord.

When the last scene of his life flashed before him, he looked back at the footprints in the sand. He noticed that many times along the path of his life there was only one set of footprints.

He also noticed that it happened at the very lowest and saddest times in his life. This really bothered him and he questioned the Lord about it.

"Lord, You said that once I decided to follow You, You'd walk with me all the way. But I have noticed that during the most troublesome times in my life, there is only one set of footprints.

"I don't understand why, when I needed You most, You would leave me."

The Lord replied,
"My son, My precious child, I love you and I would
never leave you. During your times of trial and
suffering, when you see only one set of footprints,
it was then that I carried you."

The picture below, which I share, now, with much laughter, more accurately represents my footprints journey. There was one set of footprints (His) and two deep grooves along the beach (mine). That was God having to drag me through the sand of my unbelief to where He knew I would meet truth, wholeness and hope.

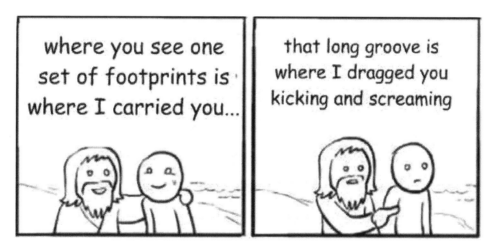

*Footprints variation

Warning

There have been so many times I've missed the clear signs of losing hope. It was like I was driving on a mountain road and seeing signs in bold print that read, "Falling Rocks Ahead", "Sharp Curve" or "Fork in Road" and not taking the necessary precautions to ensure my safety. I missed the jealousy, anger, confusion, rage and unforgiving heart signs posted all over my life. These were the warning lights on the dashboard of my soul that screamed, "Check Engine Now!" But as I said before, His voice, the voice of reason and warning can become that distant and unrecognizable Nat (natural) sound.

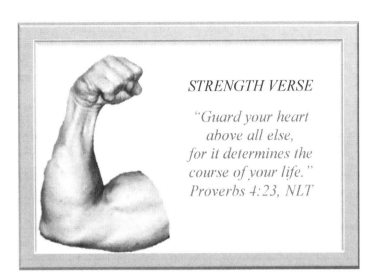

STRENGTH VERSE

"Guard your heart above all else, for it determines the course of your life."
Proverbs 4:23, NLT

I highly suggest a daily inventory of your emotions. They can become toxic when left unattended and not only destroy hope but your body as well. We will discuss this more in the chapter titled Temple Care.

STRENGTH BUILDER

1. What are some of the noises that seem to keep getting your attention?

- ☐ Jealousy
- ☐ Anger
- ☐ Confusion
- ☐ Rage
- ☐ Other _____

For further reflection, here is a list of some of the hope stoppers we encounter:

- Your past

- Unforgiveness
- Regret
- Doubt
- Negative influences/ relationships
- Pride

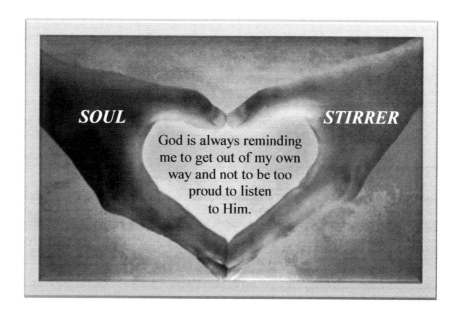

SOUL **STIRRER**

God is always reminding me to get out of my own way and not to be too proud to listen to Him.

These are what I would call hope essentials:

- God's Word
- Prayer
- Belief
- Gratitude
- Getting out of your own way
- Godly counsel
- Daily personal inventory

It's time to reignite hope in your life. Your life has left a beautiful trail of hopes and dreams, passions and pursuits. They're still waiting there to be picked up and carried victoriously to the finish line!

$2.$ Make a list of your hopes and light a huge fire in your soul believing that God has put them there for a reason. Listen to His voice and harness His hope.

MY HOPE LIST

_____	_____
_____	_____
_____	_____
_____	_____
_____	_____
_____	_____
_____	

$3.$ How did it feel to list out your hopes, dreams, passions and pursuits?

My friend Lillian once told me of the life changing hope God spoke into her heart in the midst of a suicide attempt. These words rock my soul, and I am reminded of them often.

"You don't want to die; you just don't want to hurt anymore."

She will share her amazing soul strength testimony in the chapter on Family, Relationship & Unity.

Give your life, marriage, health, workout, or whatever has died one more chance! Give God another chance and another day to reveal hope to you! Speak life into every area of struggle! I tell you the truth—there is no pill, degree or money that can give you what you truly need.

Hope is the answer and God says it's free for the asking.

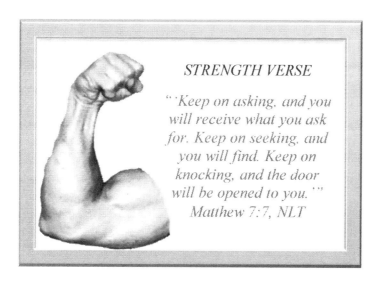

STRENGTH VERSE

"'Keep on asking, and you will receive what you ask for. Keep on seeking, and you will find. Keep on knocking, and the door will be opened to you.'"
Matthew 7:7, NLT

4. Using your hope list, write your hope story here and give it the best possible ending you can imagine.

_____

_____

_____

_____

_____

_____

_____

_____

_____

_____

_____

_____

_____

_____

_____

_____

_____

_____

CHAPTER 2

TRUST

"We cannot always trace God's hand, but we can always trust God's heart."
– Charles Spurgeon

How is your heart? Is it shattered, broken, chipped or a combination of all these? Hearts are like porcelain. They can be smashed to bits in one fall, broken over loss or lies, or chipped away at over time, losing their beauty, luster and life. Even when repaired, cracks are still visible making the heart extra fragile and sensitive to touch.

SHATTERED:

I know multitudes of you who are reading this have had your heart shattered at a tender age. As a child, my father smashed mine to bits with the hammer of his anger and bitterness. Most of us who have experienced trust-robbing abuse or neglect now consider trust like getting burned by a hot stove. After getting burned once we remember never to touch it or go near it again. Our heart becomes a thick brick wall no one can break through no matter how hard they try.

BROKEN:

Have you ever had the shock of someone suddenly walking out of a relationship with you for no apparent reason? Have you endured the sting of divorce? Such things always leave hearts and families broken. It doesn't matter how long the friendship has lasted, how great the sex is in your marriage, or how much money has been made in the business partnership. When trust is broken, so is the heart. It can be the beginning of the end. We've all suffered the loss of a parent, child, friend or even a special pet that has left a gaping break in the deepest part of our heart that we believe could never be repaired.

CHIPPED:

Throughout life our heart gets chipped away by harsh words spoken to us by others, and even ourselves. A demanding boss, or an accusing family member, or even a friend can be the one that does this. We are often our own worst enemy when it comes to chipping the heart. We speak cutting words to ourselves that we would never say to anyone else. Negative words directed at ourselves are like chisels knocking off little pieces of our heart until it becomes hard and calloused. When all of these forces are at work together, we eventually give up on trusting anyone or anything, including ourselves.

STRENGTH BUILDERS

1. What best describes the condition of your heart? Shattered? Broken? Chipped, or all of the above?

2. Write down the ways your heart has been impacted by disappointments of people in your life.

3. As you hear and consider the word trust, what are the emotions that well up inside of you?

4. What are the thoughts that come to your mind as you consider the possibility of having to take a risk and trust again?

"I TRUST NO ONE!"

That was my motto for years, and honestly it cost me dearly in my family, friendships and business. I couldn't trust people that I could see, and I definitely wouldn't trust a God that I could not see. Many times as children we see authority figures we trust, and especially parents, as God-like. After trust is broken, we carry with us a picture of that face that says, "You can't trust me," and we pin it on everyone we see, especially God, who is absolutely deserving of our trust. This can destroy a lifetime of possibilities and joy. My lack of trust stopped, limited and ruined many relationships God put in my path that could have brought deep fulfillment and led me to places I could only dream of going. Unfortunately, for many years I put the face of my earthly father on God.

A child doesn't have the strength that can hold back the power of the wounds that steal their trust. Our weapon is often an agreement we make within ourselves. I call it the "never" agreement. We may not even understand what this is at the time.

I will never allow any person to get close to me.
I will never take a risk and love someone.
I will never trust anyone but myself.
I will never believe what I hear.

As a child, the fear of someone breaking your trust again can put you in a life-long prison sentence of isolation. Over time you won't trust yourself, and you will stop making

---

We start to believe that maybe something was wrong with us...

---

decisions for your own life. We start to believe that maybe something was wrong with us and not our parents or the one who betrayed our trust. Trust-trashing words and actions leave us feeling unworthy of being loved. After being hurt or betrayed we feel like a broken toy that no one wants to play with. Our minds are like sponges that soak up the purity of truth or the poison of lies. Toxic people can fill our mind with lies that we tuck away and that eventually become our own voice that constantly whispers, *You're no good* or *You're not worthy of true love*. This is where the *can't* agreement starts:

I can't be worth loving or they wouldn't have done that to me.

I can't be a good and trustworthy person.

I can't ever do anything right.

I can't have friends because nobody can be trusted.

STRENGTH BUILDERS

1. As a child, who did you trust?

2. Who betrayed your trust?

3. What agreements did you make with yourself?

4. Have you put the face of those who have been untrustworthy on the face of others? How about God?

God tells us in Isaiah 26:3, NLT "You will keep in perfect peace all who trust in you, all whose thoughts are fixed on you!"

If your trust wounds still feel fresh you can take this verse and pin it on your heart and rehearse it in your mind daily.

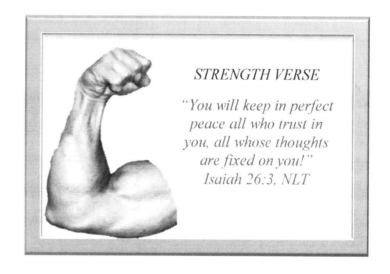

STRENGTH VERSE

"You will keep in perfect peace all who trust in you, all whose thoughts are fixed on you!"
Isaiah 26:3, NLT

If your ability to trust has been broken and you carry a deep wound, remember this and let it take root in your mind and spirit: It's not your fault. *Give any weight of guilt you may be carrying to God. He* will bear that burden and give you freedom from its grasp.

Trust is only truly restored when there is a beautiful collision of faith, hope and love.

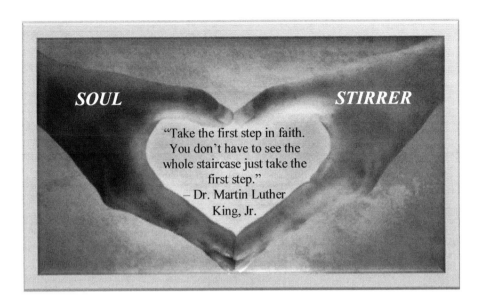

They are the triple braided rope that can pull you safely out of the pit. God is asking you to have faith that He can and wants to restore you to trust again. Dr. Martin Luther King, Jr. once said, "Take the first step in faith. You don't have to see the whole staircase just take the first step."

I want you to fill out the Trust Tracker chart on the next page. This may be difficult, but it will start the road to healing and wholeness. List anyone who betrayed your trust and also some detail of the situation. Also list anyone who held your trust and didn't betray you. This will build hope and be another tool to use in the healing process. This chart will be useful as you walk through the process of forgiveness.

Betrayed Trust (name)	Situation	

Held Trust (name)	

It's one step at a time. I must say this: Without trusting God and allowing Him to build soul strength in you, you won't be able to fully let go, forgive and trust again.

Trust is action and also a choice. A very important one! When I chose not to trust, I built a wall of muscle and alter egos around me giving me the illusion that everything was fine and I didn't have to think about trusting or forgiving. I had, so I thought, walls of my castle that could not be penetrated. It was actually a castle of sand that was eventually toppled by the waves of my past. I needed to trust!

I'm not recommending blindly trusting. That can lead to disaster, especially in intimate relationships. I would highly suggest setting up some boundaries, solid yellow lines if you will, that won't be crossed until trust is proven over a certain time period. This will give you a time space to be able to see clearly if their actions match their words.

There are also some whom you should never let into your inner circle again. They promise much and deliver little or none. There are people I had to fire out of my life because they continued to break my trust and took advantage of the grace I gave them.

STRENGTH BUILDERS

1. Write/Share how you can or cannot relate to this portion of my story.

2. Does this information give you some relief, or does it challenge you, or both? Why?

3. Make a list of those you can let back into your inner circle, and a list of those who must remain in your outer circle where relational ties must be cut off.

4. Is there someone you feel God is calling you to trust again?

Since these cuts run deep, I would highly recommend a season of seeing a Christian counselor, and also surrounding yourself with positive people of like faith. Isolation is a favorite trap of the devil.

I Swear It Won't Happen Again!

Remember this: Trust is built, not bought. It takes a lifetime to build up and a split second to destroy. One partial truth (which is actually a lie), one senseless misdeed, one secret kept can be the deal breaker for trust.

A friend of mine who loved his wife dearly became involved with another woman on Facebook. It wasn't a physical, but an emotional relationship that developed over time and was kept hidden. Eventually his wife saw the messages and was devastated, and her heart was shattered into pieces. If my friend would have developed soul strength, he would have had the ability to hear the voice of God above the voice of the flesh, and this never would have happened to them.

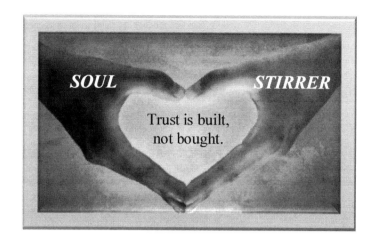

Gaining and Growing Trust Again

If you are the trust breaker, you cannot buy it back for any amount. It isn't regained by cheap promises. Action is the key that unlocks the door. Trustworthy actions over time are the bricks that build the sturdy house of restoration. If you're the one who has broken someone's trust, the burden of proof of your trustworthiness is on you! The one whose trust you broke wants to see, not hear, that you are truly and honestly sorry. You should take immediate action to show you can be trusted in the future. God can restore when you move forward in faith and repentance.

STRENGTH BUILDERS

1. Consider ways you have broken trust with others. Write them down.

2. Are you currently taking steps to bring about restoration/restored trust? If not, why not?

3. What steps do you need to take?

4. Can you remember a time when you asked for God's help and, as you followed His lead, healing happened in a relationship? Share.

Both the best and worst advice I've ever been given about trust was both short and to the point. Each was very powerful; the first in a negative way, and the latter in a positive way.

The worst was given to me by a billionaire who had every imaginable material item known to man from jet planes to mansions scattered across multiple continents. He was absolutely miserable, his children didn't respect him, and, although married, he had girlfriends all over the world. His wife was miserable as well and just endured life in an uncomfortable castle. This man was hardened. His advice was, "Trust no one." He and his wife lived this out in their marriage as well. How sad that this man didn't trust in the God who could have burned soul strength and trust into his DNA and restored all that was lost. That was a picture of me for a time. Emotional hell on earth!

The best advice was given to me by a dear friend who simply said, "Allow it." And I did! Let me tell you, there is a freedom that's like a lion being let out of his cage! God healed me and all those negative traits (bitterness, suspicion, trusting no one, isolating) started to peel off, and I finally felt comfortable in my own skin. If you refuse to trust, it's like a pecking bird that steals all of the seeds of greatness God planted in you. It's a place you don't want to stay! But as I began to choose to "Allow it," meaning, trust whatever God chose to allow in my life and follow His lead, I began to sense peace and joy and have a grateful heart for all the blessings that God provided.

In closing this chapter I will leave you with some simple, but what I believe is life changing, wisdom. Ask God into your life and into your heart and trust Him with your life. Put Him in between you and everything that is trying to steal control of your life and destroy you.

Ask God into your life and into your heart and trust Him with your life. Put Him in between you and everything that is trying to steal control of your life and destroy you.

John 10:10 says, "The thief comes only to steal and kill and destroy; I have come that they may have life, and have it to the full."

Remember this verse has two distinct parts. One of a robber and one of a redeemer! Make the Word of God your guard and keep your heart and mind safe from the thief. Experience the abundant life He is offering to you.

Psalm 9:10 says, "Those who know your name trust in you, for you, Lord, have never forsaken those who seek you."

STRENGTH BUILDERS

1. If you are hesitant in trusting God with your life, take some time to consider why—there is a reason that needs to be addressed. Think it through and write down your thoughts/hesitancies. Where are they coming from?

2. As we put our trust in Jesus, He tells us we can have life to the full—abundant life. How would that be defined in your life? What would it look like? How would things be different?

CHAPTER 3

FAMILY, RELATIONSHIP & UNITY

"A family is a place where principles are hammered and honed on the
anvil of everyday living."
– Chuck Swindoll

ALL (IS NOT WELL) IN THE FAMILY

L et's face it, when it comes to family, words like hope, trust, forgiveness and unity are like a foreign language to many of us. Like it or not, we all come from a dysfunctional family. Unfortunately, it's what we've inherited from this fallen world. But take heart—there is hope, help and healing for any family, no matter what its current state. God created the family, and it's His desire that it be healthy, loving and functional.

History Repeats

Is your family moving forward and growing strong and healthy, or is it dragging along the ball and chain of its past? One of the first items we need to pull the curtain back on is our family history. It affects much of our present. Without realizing it, most families take their cues from the culture of their past. Hurtful habits, family secrets and addictions are often handed down from one generation to the next. We model what we see and experience. A family without soul strength can't stop the generational baggage that will eventually kill, steal and destroy the love and unity it was designed by God to experience. Use this chart to take a look back on your family history. Look for clues and themes and see if they are appearing in your current family life.

See the History Repeats example and chart on pages 143 and 145.

Unity

Ronald Reagan once said that "All great change in America begins at the dinner table." How right he was! All great change *anywhere* begins in the home. Family unity is key, and the consequences of either having it or not will trickle down into all other relationships and into society itself. The family unit is under siege like never before.

For decades now the eyes of the masses have set their gaze on Hollywood's portrait of the family where adultery, substance abuse, back stabbing, and divorces of convenience have become the norm. The family values God set in place from eternity past have now become just options that are now on their way to extinction. It's painfully

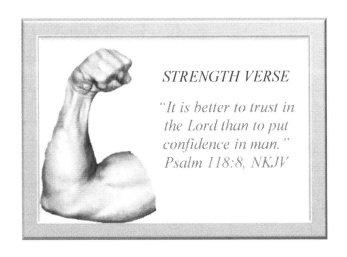

STRENGTH VERSE

"It is better to trust in the Lord than to put confidence in man."
Psalm 118:8, NKJV

clear that this system to which humankind has bowed was faulty from the very start. The broken lives and carnage of hearts and homes are countless! As families, we need to stop looking at the world for answers and stop pointing the finger of blame at each other. It's

52

time to look up at the only One who can bring order out of chaos and unity to broken families. His name is Jesus.

"It is better to trust in the Lord than to put confidence in man." – Psalm 118:8, NKJV

Is the Man of the House Home?

Much of the weight of family health lies on the back of the father. He can either plant seeds that will grow or weeds that will choke out the future of his family. Many children who have been hurt by their father never come to faith because they pin the face of their earthly father on God. A large percentage of youth who are in prison came from either a fatherless home or one where the father was emotionally absent. The world is always waiting with a counterfeit acceptance offered in gangs, cults or a substance abuse culture.

There is a thief waiting at your family's door wanting to rob you of the precious time, love and purity that would make your family strong and unified.

Consider this plea for a father who is present:

Dear Dad in the Recliner,

Long day, huh?

I bet it feels good to put your feet up.

Where is your wife?

Oh, she is tucking the children in bed.

Can I ask you something?

Why aren't you in there?

*They **need** you, Daddy.*

They find comfort in your big rough hand, smoothing their bangs off their foreheads. They love hearing your rumbly voice read them a Bible Story and a Bedtime Story. They love to hear you pray for them and their lives and futures.

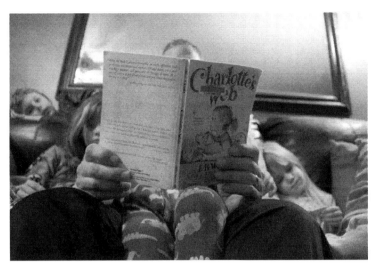

Your wife is filled with love for you, as she looks around at her little family, all together at the close of the day. Her heart swells as you kiss the children good night. She feels loved and understood when you participate in the bedtime routine.

I know you are tired, Daddy. We all are this time of the night.

***Go**.*

Go be their daddy for just a few more minutes.

As soon as they are tucked in bed, as soon as you have hugged and kissed them each twice, as soon as you have gotten them ANOTHER drink of water, after you have rubbed backs and heard precious prayers...THEN, Daddy. Then, you can go pop up the recliner, and flip on the TV or open up the newspaper.

You work hard, you deserve to relax at the end of your day; I whole heartedly agree. But, please, don't ever forget, your children will only seek you out for a short amount of years.

Then, you'll spend the rest of their lives seeking them out, and guess what?

***They won't need you anymore**.*

Not in the same way they need you now, Daddy.

You're a good Dad.

Lead your family, Daddy. Lead them straight to Jesus. Be a Holy example for those little eyes to see. They want to be just like you, so make sure you are just like HIM.

Rhythms of Life

Walking the balance beam of life is not an easy task. Work-a-holism seems to be very common in today's society. We have been fooled into thinking that more is better. More work, more money, more stuff. This is a lie from the devil and is an enemy to your family. When we live for work, or hide there for various reasons, our families starve from lack of time and attention. If 60-80 hour work weeks are your norm, you have left no margin for what your family needs most: you!

Money is important, and there are seasons of busyness when our time gets squeezed, but when the dollar, material goods and your own personal schedule have first place in your life, your family becomes a distant second. Oftentimes they're a faded memory until there is a wake-up call. I speak mainly about work here, but there are many other areas, such as hobbies, social media and friends that are competing for our attention and time. God has designed us to have a rhythm to our life. This includes family, work, rest and fun. I suggest taking a week and journaling your time. You may be surprised to see if you've left no margin for family and rest. We were created for balance, not extremes.

STRENGTH BUILDERS

1. As you consider the above sections on the family, which resonates with your family of origin? Describe how.

2. What about your current family? Share the things you are being motivated to deal with or change.

Sticks and Stones

It has been said that hurtful words are just punches thrown at the heart.

God tells us in Proverbs 18:21 that "The tongue has the power of life and death." Negative and cutting words are deadly weeds that grow rapidly and with very deep roots. Every time you speak, you scatter either seeds of love or seeds of hate. Family members, however imperfect, are a gift from God and a treasure He guards closely. Loving words, not a lashing tongue, are what they need. Children especially are living sponges, and what they soak up early in life is usually what they wring out later.

STRENGTH BUILDERS

1. Share/Write how words have been used in your life to build you up.

2. Share how they have been used to tear you down.

3. How has being built up and/or being torn down with words impacted your life decisions?

4. As you consider the many addictions in our world today, what are those that have touched you personally? Your family?

Addictions of the Heart

"For the world offers only a craving for physical pleasure, a craving for everything we see, and pride in our achievements and possessions. These are not from the Father, but are from this world." – 1 John 2:16, NLT

The slow and steady grip of pornographic images thrown at men, and women as well, has choked out many hearts that were once filled with faithful love and integrity. For the most part, men are stimulated visually and women emotionally. The devil cleverly disguises himself in provocative images that feed men's natural bent toward the visual and seductive romance scenarios that lure women's emotional nature. Each is a bait set for us to fall into his trap.

He once hid out at the corner adult store, but now has waltzed boldly into our grocery stores and right through our front door onto our computer screen. Adultery of the mind can destroy families and tear to shreds our relationship with our Heavenly Father. Social media has become a weed that is slowly choking families to death. Facebook and other media can be a dangerous lure when the heart is not fulfilled first by God, and then in marriage, if you're married. Proverbs 6:32, TLB makes it crystal clear. "The man [person] who commits adultery is an utter fool, for he destroys his own soul." Make it your lifetime goal to pursue your spouse and love him/her fully in your mind, body and spirit.

"Lord, if I ever decide to go commit adultery on my wife,
please kill me on the way there."

"Therefore what God has joined together, let no one separate." – Mark 10:9

Search the Scriptures to gain the soul strength that will build and keep a faithful heart by studying what God has to say about faithfulness. Someone told me about a very bold prayer a man once said at a Promise Keepers event: "Lord, if I ever decide to go commit adultery on my wife, please kill me on the way there." I believe his heart was stirred by God's stern words about the consequences of breaking the covenant of marriage.

Technology gods

Twenty years ago who would have thought that a little device we could hold in our hand would command our attention more than family, friends, work and even God. Text messages, games, email, phone calls and a myriad of other attention grabbers are all at the tip of our fingers 24/7. Many people are driving, walking, meeting or having dinner together with their heads bobbing up and down as they look for the next message or call to come in. This, I believe, has become a full blown addiction for many and is causing the breakdown and sometimes the break-up of families and friendships. The only one we should be available for everyday all day is God. Being distracted makes us unable to hear the voice that can direct, comfort, and lead us. I am not against technology. Much of what I do relies on it, but I'm seeing it as a growing tool the enemy is using to take us away from what we really need, which is our time and relationship with God and with our families. We can't text ourselves to deeper relationships with family and friends. It's just not how our Creator designed us. Try writing a hand written letter to someone or meeting with a friend instead of texting 20 times. There is a richness in experiencing people and developing relationships that technology can never match. Before you answer the next series of questions, know that I understand that modern work requires a lot of social media and text communication and sometimes there truly is no time to meet with people, but I want you to be honest about this because it matters to your relationship with God and others.

STRENGTH BUILDERS

1. Describe how pornography has impacted your life (either personally or through someone else).

2. If pornography is a personal struggle, what steps are you taking to guard your heart against this trap?

3. How much time do you spend each week on social media, texting and computer (non-work related)?

4. If these activities are consuming too much of your time, what are some ways you could cut back and make more time for prayer, developing relationships and simply hearing the voice of God?

5. What are your feelings about technology and how it affects your life?

6. How would your life and family look if activities in your life were simplified?

Seeds

Time with your family is a seed that grows for eternity. The good memories I have about my family are when we were all together sharing, laughing and loving. Do you have a family prayer time? Do you have meals together as often as possible? Do you take vacations together? These are all must-haves for a solid foundation of a strong family with love and unity.

Servant leadership. Your family, not the church, needs to be your first ministry. Live what you preach! Whether you know it or not, you are being watched all the time. Immediate and extended family are all affected by your words and actions. Devote time to the needs of your wife or husband and children. Find out what those needs are by asking. And for singles, you

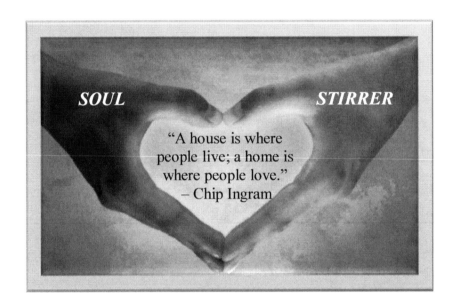

SOUL STIRRER

"A house is where people live; a home is where people love."
– Chip Ingram

can do the same with your extended family or spiritual family. Have family time to hear the victories and defeats of their day. Be the encourager and bring them to a higher level of living. Make your home a safe place where everyone can share all that is on their heart without fear of criticism or judgment. Joy and oneness should be the norm.

Faith. The solid foundation of faith keeps a family strong in all seasons of life. Families without faith will never reach their full potential. Answers to life's problems can't come from the world's wisdom. Society is living proof that without rightly placed faith there is failure.

Mothers

Meekness = power under control.

There is no power and love like that of a mother. Even with the heavy burden of my dad being an alcoholic and womanizer, my mother managed to make an unsafe place safe. She showed consistent positive behavior in an environment that was being led by a divided spirit. Her saying, "This too shall pass" and "The sun will shine again" ring in my ears to this day. This five foot tall giant of God's love was the knife in the heart of the dysfunction that could have destroyed our family as a whole.

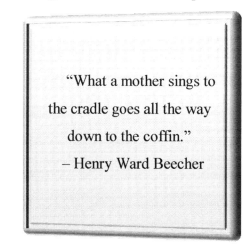

"What a mother sings to the cradle goes all the way down to the coffin."
– Henry Ward Beecher

Mothers, however, can have a profound negative impact on each member of the family as well by criticizing words, shutting down or picking a favorite child. Mothers, remember your heart is the bed on which your family can safely lie.

Mothers, as well as all of us, should constantly consider the impact of their choices. Listen to this story.

Dear Mom on the iPhone,

I see you over there on the bench, messing on your iPhone. It feels good to relax a little while your kids have fun in the sunshine, doesn't it? You are doing a great job with your kids, you work hard, you teach them manners, have them do their chores.

*But Momma, let me tell you what you **don't** see right now....*

Your little girl is spinning round and round, making her dress twirl. She is such a little beauty queen already, the sun shining behind her hair. She keeps glancing your way to see if you are watching her.

You aren't.

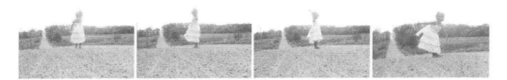

Your little boy keeps shouting, "Mom, MOM watch this!" I see you acknowledge him, barely glancing his way.

He sees that too. His shoulders slump, but only for a moment, as he finds the next cool thing to do.

Now you are pushing your baby in the swing. She loves it! Cooing and smiling with every push. You don't see her though, do you? Your head is bent, your eyes on your phone as you absently push her swing.

Talk to her. Tell her about the clouds, Mommy. The Creator who made them. Tickle her tummy when she comes near you and enjoy that baby belly laugh that leaves far too quickly.

Put your eyes back on your prize...Your kids.

*Show them that **they** are the priority. Wherever you are, be ALL there. I am not saying it's not ok to check in on your phone, but it's a time-sucker: User Beware!*

Play time at the park will be over before you know it.

The childhood of your children will be gone before you know it.

They won't always want to come to the park with you, Mommy. They won't always spin and twirl to make their new dress swish, they won't always call out, "WATCH ME!"

There will come a point when they stop trying, stop calling your name, stop bothering to interrupt your phone time.

Because they know...

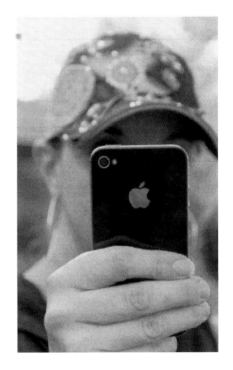

You've shown them, all these moments, that the phone is more important than they are. They see you looking at it while waiting to pick up brother from school, during playtime, at the dinner table, at bedtime....

I know that's not true, Mommy.

I know your heart says differently.

But your kids can't hear your words, Mommy. Your actions are screaming way too loudly.

*May our eyes rest upon those we love, first and foremost, and may **everything else** fall away in the wonderful, noisy, sticky-fingered glory of it all.*

Children are looking for examples from both mother and father. They want to see us live out our faith. Here is an excellent example of just that. Not long after my divorce, when my daughters were 15 and 13, I decided to have them sign a purity code. My younger daughter agreed but my older daughter hesitated saying, "Daddy, this just shows you don't trust me." As she was about to reluctantly sign, she put the pen down and walked into the library with the agreement. I didn't have a clue as to what she was doing until she appeared with another copy in her hand, one for me to sign. This was such a precious moment for me. It was also a stark reminder of how much our children want to see our beliefs put into action. Our influence and actions are the school teachers of their heart. The fact is, many children will marry, for better or worse, someone just like their parents.

STRENGTH BUILDERS

1. Share/Write out the positive seeds that have been planted in your life from your biological and/or spiritual families.

2. Have there been "seed" robbers? What/Who were they?

3. Share/Write about your relationship with your father.

4. Share/Write about your relationship with your mother.

The Exhausted Family

Without soul strength, family will burn out on its own power. God will let us do it on our own until we're completely out of gas and turn to Him. The roots must be deep in God's design or there will be a break down. Overloaded work schedules and going to every function that comes up leaves little time for personal family growth. Families need to communicate daily. It's how we get to know each other at the deepest level.

Investing time is not the same as spending it. Take a day vacation from technology. When it feels like you can't get off the treadmill of life, do the wise thing and stop, drop and pray! Give it to Him immediately and seek His will. Quit asking God to bless what you're doing; find out what God is doing and follow that because it's already blessed. God gave us our families and it's wise to invest in them. The return on this investment is beyond measure. It's also extremely important for husbands and wives to have alone time for sharing, fun and closeness. This creates a deep bond, not only for spouses, but a bond that has a profound effect on the family as well.

STRENGTH BUILDERS

1. What does your weekly schedule look like? Are you allowing margin?

2. Is there time for deep connection in the relationships you have—especially in your family?

Turn to page 141 in the back of this book. Use this simple chart to make a schedule for the week. If you fail to plan, you plan to fail; it's as simple as that. We all should have a healthy rhythm to our life. It's really all about proper balance and order. This will take some trial and error to perfect, but it will be well worth the effort, and it will also save you a lot of frustration and also keep you from the all-too-common burnout and neglect stages that most are accustomed to calling "normal." As you fill out this chart, I want you to look for areas in your life that are out of balance, extreme or neglected. I would also like you to take a week and track your time to see where you and your family can prioritize time together.

Unpack Your Bags

We all have baggage from our past, and it can be the silent and sneaky killer of our relationships if we don't deal with it. As I've said to many couples that I've counseled before marriage, "Know exactly what is in each other's carry-on luggage before you board the flight."

The reason why pre-marital counseling is so vitally important is that we need to get to know each other's hurts, habits and hang-ups to get an understanding of how to meet each other's needs and deal with remnants of the past.

The foundation is cracked, the roof is leaking and the carpet is soaked! This may be an accurate metaphor of the current state of your family. Even if this is your family portrait right now, don't give up. God is the Creator and Rescuer of families. I know this first hand! Your Creator is offering you a relationship, and with that, the power of soul strength to hear His plan of recovery.

STRENGTH BUILDERS

1. Have you ever considered the baggage you might have from other relationships? Or baggage from your family of origin?

2. What baggage do you need to unpack to move forward in a relationship/marriage?

One giant first step is to do an inventory of our feelings and responses to daily life. Reactive living ends up taking us all over the map, putting our emotions in control, and ends up producing chaotic and anxious living. Proactive living on the other hand sets the course ahead of time so that we're not swayed by circumstance or withered by the wearing of daily obstacles.

We must learn from the past. When we do an inventory, we get a clear indication of things to change in our lives. Then we can take the brush of God's grace and forgiveness and start to paint a new and beautiful picture of our family life. Family is a unit, and we must grow through our issues, not get trapped in them. God truly meant for the family to have joy, and for that joy to come from Him. A family is also a place of growth where we become more like Jesus, bearing the fruit of His spirit.

Ecclesiastes 4:12, NLT says, "A person standing alone can be attacked and defeated, but two can stand back-to-back and conquer. Three are even better, for a triple-braided cord [God/parents/children] is not easily broken." To safeguard your family's future, take time to talk over the issues that everyone faced that day, find out if there are needs that aren't being met, and encourage one another. This will help ensure success in the home. Look ahead and get a read on anything that is coming up in the future that you have control over. Plan ahead and keep family in its proper place. Do something about issues at home as soon as you can—don't wait. Procrastination is a sharp tool the enemy uses to carve a deep division between family members.

Proverbs 3:21-23, ERV says, "My son, don't ever let wisdom out of your sight. Hold on to wisdom and careful planning. They will bring you a long life filled with honor. As you go through life, you will always be safe and never fall."

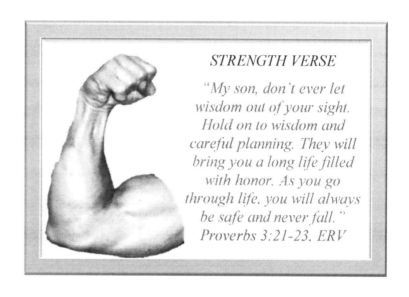

STRENGTH VERSE

"My son, don't ever let wisdom out of your sight. Hold on to wisdom and careful planning. They will bring you a long life filled with honor. As you go through life, you will always be safe and never fall."
Proverbs 3:21-23, ERV

Single or married, having a community of healthy friends is extremely important to your emotional health and well-being. We need relationships that are a safe place to be ourselves and where we won't feel judged no matter what we've done or are going through. Again we need healing from the past via soul strength to take a faith risk and develop close friendships.

I went through a long season in my life where I was a lone wolf. I used to say, "I don't need *anyone* to make me happy. If someone wants to join me, I will share my happiness

We need to start each day by asking God to reveal who we are in Him and go out into the world as His child, loving who we are, and also giving His love to everyone He has placed in our lives.

with them." Actually I was terrified of getting hurt again by giving my heart away. I would retreat and isolate by living in my own private world. In public I would often wear a mask and be the person others thought I should be. Wearing a mask is a prison we stay in that keeps us from being the person God wants us to become. We need to start each day by asking God to reveal who we are in Him and go out into the world as His child, loving who we are, and also giving His love to everyone He has placed in our lives. As it has been said, value people and use things, don't value things and use people.

Our Spiritual Family

Hebrews 10:25, NLT says, "And let us not neglect our meeting together, as some people do, but encourage one another, especially now that the day of his return is drawing near."

There is one last family that we shouldn't forget, and that is vital to our life. That is our spiritual family. God intended the church family (His body) to reflect His unity, which is the trinity (Father, Son and Holy Spirit). Church should be a place of preparation and encouragement so that we can go out and reach the lost and needy world with His love firmly planted in our hearts. Fellowship and accountability is vital to our spiritual health and growth as Christ followers. The family of God should do life together, not just say hi and bye on Sundays.

We need an up, in and out lifestyle. Looking up to Him, looking into our own hearts, having deep intimate community, and reaching out to serve and reach the world around us, whether on our own block or around the world. In short, we need to do life together, encouraging and praying for each other, meeting the needs of our spiritual family and our community. The church should look like the picture we see in Scripture. Acts chapter 2:42-47 describes believers as ones who worship together, share all they have with each other and those in need, eating together, giving money to those without, and praising God and enjoying fellowship. If you're just attending a church service on Sunday and then going about your week, you are robbing yourself of a blessing God wants you to have with His family.

Many of us, single or married, have never had a good role model in our lives. We may have never had a biological family we could count on, let alone a church family. There is

The family of God should do life together....

something very special that God did in my life and He will do in yours too. He will re-parent us by sending spiritual mothers or fathers as guides and faithful role models. Paul Bersche was a spiritual father to me. God sent him as a gift and a compass for my life. He gave me renewed hope and the ability to trust in a father figure again. I now experience a healthy biological and spiritual family. God wants to restore all that the enemy has stolen from your heart and your family.

STRENGTH BUILDERS

1. Are you living a "reactive" life or a "proactive" life? How?

2. Can you think of an individual who was not your parent, but who has been in your life and provided nurture or guidance when you needed it? Share.

3. Are you connected to a spiritual family? If so, describe how this has been significant in your life. If not, why not?

My prayer is that a new norm for you will be having a functional and healthy family.

As we conclude this chapter, I want to leave you with some ideas you can write on a paper and in your heart. These are simple yet profound seeds that will spark your family to grow in deeper love and unity.

- Speak life. We need to inventory ourselves about the words we speak to our family and friends. Are they building up or tearing down? Even in conflict we can still speak words of peace and life. Here's a great idea. Try to catch your family doing something good, and then speak words of encouragement to them.

- Hold moments. There are many moments of our family life that we rush by not realizing our Creator has given us a "God sighting" and wants us to stop and soak them up in our heart. Hold these moments dear because you can't get them back.

- Give out by being selfless, and give up by letting God be God. He is able! Putting others first in a healthy way gives joy in the depths of our being like almost nothing else. By giving up trying to control all situations, it gives us the chance to see God work all things out for His glory and our good.

- Random acts of kindness. Surprise your family and friends with an unexpected favor or a gift they weren't expecting. You will touch a deep part of their heart.

- Be present and attentive when you're with your family. Don't be distracted by the phone or other electronic devices when spending time with loved ones. They need your full attention. As I said before, the voice of God can easily be drowned out by distractions. Take a technology vacation and spend some time just communicating. God made us for relationship.

- Marriage is a covenant not a contract. A contract is usually an obligation for a limited time. A family and marriage covenant is forever. Honoring marriage as a covenant is God's way and His will, and it will make a family strong.

- Life by The Book. God's Word is a weapon of mass instruction! And of course mass destruction to our enemy, if it is obeyed. Knowing and living His Word will bring your family from the prison to the palace.

- Serve your family. There are plenty of books and seminars about leadership, but very few on serving. Serve your family with a humble heart. Find out what their needs are and meet those needs with a committed and joyful heart. Make Jesus your primary example of a servant's heart. He served as He led.

The following story is an example of how God can take a life that was programmed to fail and turn it into a powerful tool for furthering His kingdom. Luke 18:27, NLT says, "What is impossible from a human perspective is possible with God."

Lillian's Living Hope Story

I grew up in a very painful environment. My father was an alcoholic and we (my mom and three sisters) never knew what we would encounter on a daily basis. I lived in fear and witnessed a lot of physical abuse. I also endured much emotional and verbal abuse. I was very insecure, although you'd never suspect it from the outside. Because of our family dysfunction,

I was never encouraged to dream, have goals or develop my life. I internalized a lot of shame and didn't see any hope for the future.

I allowed this to lead me to find my comfort in drugs and alcohol. By age seventeen, I had dropped out of high school and was married. My husband was also an addict. By my late twenties, the baggage of my family history and my addictions had become a weight far too heavy to carry.

I was a broken woman on the verge of divorce; and I was alone (since everyone pretty much disowned me because of my behavior). I was defeated and totally disgusted with myself. It was then that I decided that the only way of escape was suicide. As I drank and took every pill I could find, I wrote letters to family and friends saying good-bye.

What I saw in the mirror was pitiful and hopeless, but that wasn't what God saw. He had another plan. It was in my desperation that He met me. I know it was His voice of strength saying to me, "You don't want to die; you just don't want to hurt anymore."

I made myself throw up again and again. It took me three days to recover. Once I came out of that, I thought of my dad, who by now had been modeling sobriety for seven years. We would sit and talk for hours about his amazing experience with God and how he had a brand new peace and purpose. This took me back to my childhood and reminded me of our wonderful loving neighbors who took me to Sunday School and Vacation Bible School until I was ten years old. It was there that God actually started to lay a foundation in my heart, but one that He would have to dig up after many years of abuse and addiction.

I attended a church service one week after talking to my father, and it was there I met Jesus Christ so very powerfully. I never took another drink again. By God's grace and the strength of His Holy Spirit, I was able to get whole and healthy.

I reconciled with my family and started leading addiction support groups. God, by His amazing grace, made a ministry out of my misery. For

25 years now, God has allowed me to lead others from their hurts, habits and hang-ups to knowing Jesus, the true healer and God that saves.

I am now blessed with a godly marriage to a husband who was also delivered from the grip of addiction. We are partners with God in reaching out to the depressed, lonely, hopeless and addicted through a support group ministry called LifeCare that I formed several years ago.

I am living the abundant life God promised! It's not problem and pain free, but fulfilled and joy filled from the inside out! I can't imagine doing anything more fulfilling than living for Christ and seeing others transformed by His love.

Jesus wants to turn your life around no matter what the past or present circumstances. He is able! I am a walking billboard of His promise and unconditional love!

STRENGTH BUILDERS

1. Write out the seeds (e.g., acts of kindness, encouraging words, commitment, being fully attentive) that you need to begin to plant in your relationships.

2. Respond to the story you just read. Are there things in Lillian's life that resonate with you and your situation, current or past?

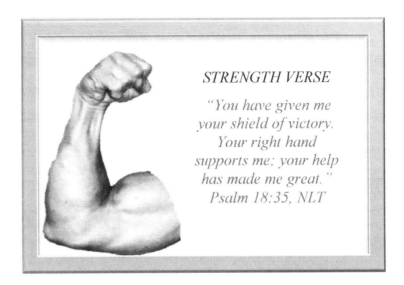

STRENGTH VERSE

*"You have given me
your shield of victory.
Your right hand
supports me; your help
has made me great."*
Psalm 18:35, NLT

CHAPTER 4

FORGIVENESS

"To forgive is to set a prisoner free and discover that the prisoner was you."

– Philip Yancey

W hat is forgiveness?

The core of forgiveness is releasing someone of an emotional debt that they owe. It's a pardon and cancellation of that debt without condition. This does not mean, however, that we put ourselves back into a dangerous or harmful situation.

Forgiveness and Reconciliation

We often confuse forgiveness and reconciliation. As an overview, forgiveness takes one and reconciliation takes two. The difference is that reconciliation requires a change in behavior in the other person, as well as their willingness to reconcile. Forgiveness takes place vertically, between you and God, and does not require any action from the one who offended you. You can forgive someone without the relationship having to be restored. Reconciliation is horizontal and requires action from both the one who was offended and the offender.

Forgiving someone does not mean what they did to you was okay, and it does not require you to let someone back into your life. Without a change on their part, reconciling may not happen.

Why Forgive?

- If you're a Christ follower, God commands it. Matthew 6:15, NLT says, "'But if you refuse to forgive others, your Father will not forgive your sins.'"

- It is a reflection of our Creator. Romans 5:8, NLT says, "But God showed his great love for us by sending Christ to die for us while we were still sinners."

- When you forgive, you take ammunition away from the enemy of your soul, the devil himself. When you don't forgive, he thrives and waves the flag of victory over you.

- You empower yourself to live free and are able to have healthy relationships.

- It will bring spiritual and emotional health, as well as physical health, to your body. It's like a medicine that can restore you to wholeness on every level.

- Forgiveness frees you from being under the power and control of another person or circumstance.

Forgiveness Frauds

Real forgiveness is impossible when we try to use are own formulas to make it happen. There are three that are very common and ones I used much throughout my life.

- **Conditional**

  I will only forgive if…. With this formula, we usually set the bar very high for the other person to jump through. If they don't meet our standards, we will not forgive.

o **Avoidance**

Ignore won't restore. Sometimes we think that ignoring the hurt that comes from an offense will make it go away because we have heard all of our lives that time will heal all wounds. Ignoring your pain from being hurt will not bring about forgiveness but instead plants and waters the seeds of resentment and bitterness. For years, I thought I forgave my father and others for offenses and pain they

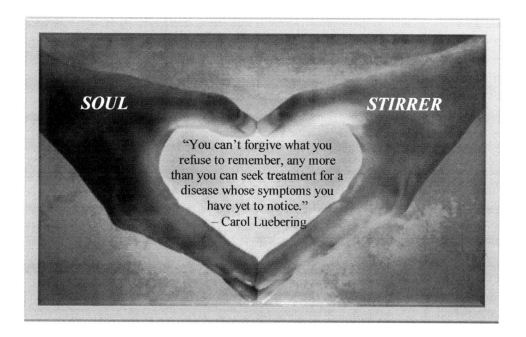

SOUL   STIRRER

"You can't forgive what you refuse to remember, any more than you can seek treatment for a disease whose symptoms you have yet to notice."
– Carol Luebering

caused me, but what I was really doing was avoiding the pain. I medicated myself with hours upon hours in the gym. I looked healthy on the outside, but on the inside, I was being eaten alive.

o **Forgiveness in Mind Only**

We can think we forgive, but if it's only in our mind and not our heart, the wound will never heal. Without heart forgiveness, we will get sad, angry or resentful every time the offense is thought of or mentioned. A song, place or even a smell can well up memories of the hurt and take us right back to the offense. Often when this happens, we immediately try to fill our thoughts and our lives with anything that will deaden the pain and hurt. It's not a healthy or safe place to hide when the memory comes to call. Unhealed pain is often the birthplace for addiction.

You've probably tried one or more of the above methods at least once if not multiple times. Maybe they've been a life theme for you. I know they were for me.

These all have one thing in common. You are using your own power to attempt to forgive, and that's not enough. It took me fifteen years to truly forgive my dad, and that was only after I had a relationship with Jesus. His power alone gives the strength to forgive!

The devil wants you to stay in a constant state of unforgiveness and resentment. He loves when you feel but don't heal. A great example of this is what Chris Thurman used in his book, *The Lies We Believe*: You take a 5¢ offense and put a $500 value on it. A 5¢ offense is a small offense that could typically be overlooked easily (e.g., your friend parking in your driveway when you'd prefer he park in the street), and a $500 offense would be something typically very difficult to move past (e.g., infidelity by your spouse).

When you have 5¢ offenses where you put a $500 value on it, these offenses build up over a lifetime and "suddenly" we have a million dollars' worth in our unforgiveness bank. At this point it feels impossible to forgive. This will eventually cause a tidal wave of destruction that will, sadly, wreck many of our relationships. God commands us to forgive, and when he commands something, He gives us the power to do it. It's for our benefit and for our freedom and wholeness that we are to release these debts. My life changed dramatically when I was able to (through a relationship with Jesus) surrender the heavy burden of not forgiving those who caused me pain and shame.

STRENGTH BUILDERS

1. What are some of the methods you have used to try to forgive those who have hurt you?

2. Have you tried any of those that I listed? Share/Write about those times and use specifics.

In order to forgive from the heart, you have to rid yourself of the ways you have attempted it and failed. Looking at those specific instances will help you in that process.

Consequences of Unforgiveness

Remember there are *always* consequences to unforgiveness.

1. **Physical**. Fear and anger are almost always involved in unforgiveness. Physically, when you have fear and anger, your body releases cortisol, which is your body's fight or flight hormone. When you don't forgive, you create stress, and then a constant flow of cortisol is released, causing something called homosysteine. This creates an inflammation in the body. It is like keeping the gas pedal of your car pushed to the floor. After so long, the engine blows. Long term inflammation has been linked to cancer, heart disease and a host of other life-threatening diseases.

2. **Mental**. You will become double-minded and distracted. Your focus can't be on two things at once. If you continue to focus on the person who offended you, you will be unable to think clearly in other important areas of your life that need attention. The enemy's battle ground is in your mind. He wants to claim it as his territory.

3. **Spiritual**. The spiritual implications of not forgiving causes severe static in the communication line between you and God. You will no longer experience the

power of soul strength that comes from being able to hear the guiding voice of your Creator. We were made to experience inner joy and freedom that does not come from external circumstances, but it comes from the very presence of the Lord living within us. Unforgiveness is a lock that keeps the doors of heaven closed in our lives. Plain and simple, it's a device the devil uses to bring division, bitterness and hatred among God's children. For the Christian, forgiving is *not* a suggestion or something to try if we're in the mood; it's a command to follow. Colossians 3:13, NLT says, "Make allowance for each other's faults, and forgive anyone who offends you. Remember, the Lord forgave you, so you must forgive others." Unforgiveness is in violation of the very foundation of our belief, the cross of Christ. A person who forgives is letting the power of our forgiving God flow through him or her. There is a joyful freedom that allows you to love more deeply and draw closer to others.

4. **Relational/Family**. I have counseled countless families who have been split for decades because of unforgiveness over small and large offenses, and sometimes they can't even recall the offense that caused them not to forgive. I've also seen the pain and regret in the hearts of many who, at the funerals and grave sites of loved ones (both family and estranged friendships), wished they had allowed the seeds of forgiveness a chance to grow. The acid of a hard heart can quickly dissolve relationships that otherwise could have given lifetime enrichment and left a loving legacy of unity and oneness that God created families and friendships to have.

Below, fill in the name of the person who offended you, when the offense occurred and what happened.

(Who)_____ hurt me (when)_____ (how)_____.

(Who)_____ hurt me (when)_____ (how)_____.

(Who)_____ hurt me (when)_____ (how)_____.

(Who)_____ hurt me (when)_____ (how)_____.

(Who)_____ hurt me (when)_____ (how)_____.

Will the Real Forgiveness Please Stand Up?

We've seen examples of false forgiveness and what happens when we try to forgive with our own might. Now let's look at three foundations necessary for the forgiveness process to take place.

- **Feel** – We all feel all the time. When we are hurt, our emotions can run wild and even be felt in our physical bodies. God gave us feelings and they are good, but they are also indicators of something else going on, something beneath the surface. We need to look under the hood, so to speak, and find out where the cause of the feeling *really* came from. Go to a quiet place so you won't have the distractions that come with familiar surroundings.

- **Deal** – It is a must that we take a time of personal reflection and work through the feelings and memories of offenses, taking account of the damage done to us. Using a journal to pour out the feelings of past hurt and anger is very helpful. You can look back on the

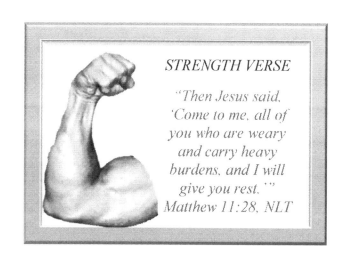

STRENGTH VERSE

"Then Jesus said, 'Come to me, all of you who are weary and carry heavy burdens, and I will give you rest.'"
Matthew 11:28, NLT

progress you've made and also see themes and patterns reflected in how you've dealt with hurt.

- **Heal** – This is where a very important word comes into play: surrender. Surrender means bringing that person and the offense before God, along with all the honest emotions you are experiencing about the offender, and trusting God to bring about the change of heart of both you and the one who hurt you. This may take time and not feel natural, but it will be worth it. You may need to express anger, tears, sorrow or many other emotions. God wants you to be free by taking that burden off your back. The weight is way too heavy to carry alone.

  In Matthew 11:28, NLT Jesus says, "'Come to me, all of you who are weary and carry heavy burdens, and I will give you rest.'"

Forgiving the Unforgivable

Harnessing the power of soul strength is the only way to be victorious here. Things that might have been done to us are so horrific and detestable that it may seem we can't live with the memory of them. God is able to take you back to that place of hurt and reveal His truth about the experience. He alone can make your heart whole again and able to fully forgive.

Forgiven but Not Forgotten

Here is the place to harness the power of soul strength. Our minds have an endless capacity to store memories and can be triggered to recall memories in a split second. We may never forget what happened to us, but by choosing the power of soul strength, the memories will no longer be able to master our mind.

"Forgiveness does not erase the bitter past. A healed memory is not a deleted memory. Instead, forgiving what we cannot forget creates a new way to remember. We change the memory of our past into a hope for our future." (Flanigan)

Forgiving Self

Throughout our lifetime we can stack up much shame, guilt and regret. Forgiving ourselves often seems like a "get off the hook" scheme because we feel like we must pay back and reconcile every offense we've made. Someone once told me, "Peter, if God forgave you, who are you to say you can't forgive yourself?" Self-hatred and self-punishment are not God's design for you. Understand and accept your imperfections, and don't hold yourself to a higher standard than even God does. Dwelling on your past wrongs and counting on your own reasoning will fog your thinking. God is not dwelling on your past, no matter how bad, but He is calling you to have child-like faith and simply believe His promise of forgiveness. He is not asking for performance and perfection as we often ask of ourselves, but He is persuading you to surrender. If you're at the end of your rope of self-strength, just let go and fall gently into the arms of a forgiving God who loves you unconditionally. Your past mistakes don't define who you are; God's unconditional love and forgiveness do. You cannot be whole and emotionally healthy (for yourself or anybody else) until you've forgiven yourself. I can't stress this enough! Your whole inner being can be at stake here.

Forgiving Someone Who is No Longer Alive

In many cases the person you need to forgive has passed on from this life. Although

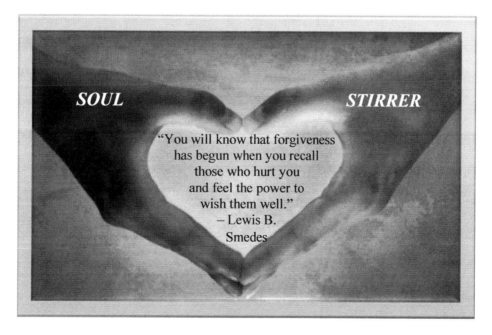

SOUL STIRRER

"You will know that forgiveness has begun when you recall those who hurt you and feel the power to wish them well."
– Lewis B. Smedes

communication with them is no longer possible, you can have the freedom of forgiving them. Try writing them a letter from your heart, releasing them from the debt. You can throw it out or keep it as a reminder when the debt seed tries to plant itself in your mind again. Place a chair opposite of you and envision the person sitting and listening attentively. You can do the same at a grave site where it's just God, you and the memory of the hurt. Pour your heart out before God and the person. If there is still anger present, let it out and then give yourself permission to let it flow into forgiveness. Before you explore these options, ask God to meet you at the very place and time of the hurt. It is there that He will lovingly reveal His perspective and gladly give you the soul strength of a forgiving heart.

How Will You Know that You've Truly Forgiven?

You will know that you've truly forgiven when the powerful feelings of revenge, bitterness or sadness are greatly reduced or even non-existent when memories of that person or hurt surface. There will be a steady peace that was not present before.

STRENGTH BUILDERS

1. What part of this section in the chapter has challenged you?

2. Write out the information or highlight the parts that were new for you. Spend some time contemplating it and write out how this new information changes things for you as it relates to forgiveness and reconciliation.

The power of looking in and up becomes the core of your power to forgive. Ask God to remind you of His grace and sacrifice that made the forgiveness of your own sin possible. This is the spiritual fuel that fills you with the strength to pray for the well-being of those who wronged you and also to fully accept the forgiveness God freely offers in His Son, Jesus. This will also give you the joy of offering mercy and forgiving quickly before the enemy has a chance to cultivate the ground for resentment and bitterness.

Colossians 3:13, NLT says, "Make allowance for each other's faults, and forgive anyone who offends you. Remember, the Lord forgave you, so you must forgive others."

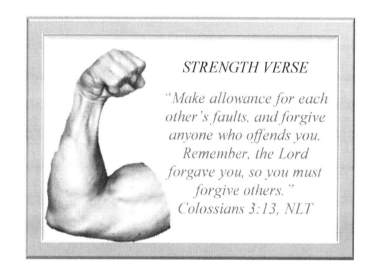

STRENGTH VERSE

"Make allowance for each other's faults, and forgive anyone who offends you. Remember, the Lord forgave you, so you must forgive others."
Colossians 3:13, NLT

One of the most important things I've ever done is relinquish the debt of my dad. When I did this, it seemed like every area of my life went from dark to light. Not only will forgiving bless you, but it will bless all others in your life as well. Our actions show our trust in either God or ourselves. Unforgiveness is all about self. Forgiveness is about God. Be wise and make it about Him. He alone gives us the power and peace to forgive.

Asking For Forgiveness

When we are the one who has hurt or offended, we need to ask forgiveness with a few things in mind. We must understand that most times this will be a process. Action always needs to accompany asking forgiveness—our behavior needs to change. Talk without action is cheap and will prove that you are not sincere. I've seen God work literal miracles in relationships when there is true repentance and sacrificial efforts to bring about forgiveness and reconciliation. God designed us for relationships. Unity and peace are His plan for us.

Whether having to forgive or be forgiven, there can be a deep battle. The other person may not forgive you, and outside influences from others can hinder the reconciliation process. I remind you, there are unseen forces of evil at work in and around us. They battle for control of our mind and heart. On this earth there is spiritual warfare. God is sovereign, and He will give us victory and peace even in the midst of this raging battle.

Ephesians 6:12, NIV says, "For our struggle is not against flesh and blood, but against the rulers, against the authorities, against the powers of this dark world and against the spiritual forces of evil in the heavenly realms."

Forgiveness and reconciliation are really God's story. On the cross below, the arrows that are pointing up and down indicate forgiveness (which is between us and God), and the arrows pointing side to side indicate reconciliation (which, by God's grace, can happen between us and others).

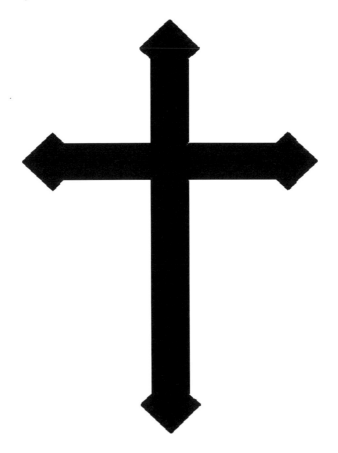

True forgiveness comes only by way of the cross. Jesus gives forgiveness and reconciliation to all who ask.

Psalm 103:10-12 (NLT),
"He does not punish us for all our sins;
　he does not deal harshly with us, as we deserve.
For his unfailing love toward those who fear him
　is as great as the height of the heavens above the earth.
He has removed our sins as far from us
　as the east is from the west."

I want to leave this chapter with a powerful living hope story of Kelly Hawkins, an author friend of mine, that includes most of what we've covered in this chapter. It's a story of abuse, pain and shame that led to the narrow but beautiful road of redemption and unconditional forgiveness.

　　Growing up, I felt a lack of adequate attention and affection, which left me with an emptiness and hunger to be filled. When an uncle started giving me lots of attention and affection, it felt refreshing to me, and the emptiness began to dissipate.

　　It wasn't long, though, before those interactions became unhealthy, and I was sexually abused by my uncle from ages 12-14. I stayed silent though. I kept wanting to feel his "love" again (the life-giving attention and affection I experienced in the beginning), and I didn't want to feel like the "cause" of breaking up a family if I did say something. So I kept the silence that my uncle demanded.

　　Eventually, all the attention stopped and I felt even emptier, and rejected as well. I was 18 or 19 when I first talked about my uncle's interactions with me, but I didn't even identify what had happened as abuse at that time—I just considered it a "bad relationship." As I learned more about sexual abuse, I realized what that experience really was.

Eventually, I began to look at the things my uncle gave me, as well as what he stole from me that he could never give back. Initially, he did give me healthy attention and affection where I lacked it. But he quickly began to steal from me. He stole my innocence and purity—not just physically, but also emotionally, relationally and even spiritually as he changed the way I saw God. He stole my close relationship with my aunt. He stole what could have been a healthy uncle/niece relationship that could have nurtured me with safety and security. Instead, he stole safety and security from me.

I knew these were things he could never repay; in fact, he wasn't even aware of what his actions actually stole from me. It made me think of Jesus on the cross when He said, "'Father, forgive them, for they do not know what they are doing.'" (Luke 23.34, NIV)

Because I was able to see and understand Jesus' example, I was able to forgive my uncle—to let go of what he owed me and realize that Jesus could take my loss and do something good and beautiful with it. He promises in Romans 8.28 that He will use ALL things for good when we choose to love Him and trust Him.

When my uncle called me a couple years later to ask for forgiveness, and I told him I had already forgiven him, I could say it peacefully and with compassion because of what God had already done in my heart to give me freedom. My uncle, however, had still been in bondage to his sin that had been internally destroying him.

Twenty years later, I found myself struggling to forgive "smaller", day-to-day offenses and live in wholeness. By this time, I had been a Christian for 38 years. God had done a lot of refining in my life, and I didn't see much in me that was wrong or offensive to God. I felt like I was doing okay, but still had trouble forgiving those "smaller" offenses.

I knew I had some underlying anxiety issues that were not readily visible to others, so still, I appeared okay on the surface, but God began to deal with those issues.

At first, some relational insecurities began to surface. I quickly told God we needed to deal with this. I knew that the insecurities would cause relational harm if they were to completely surface and I was to act out on them. So I told God I was ready for those to be healed and I would do whatever it took to get that healing.

It sounded like a good plan to me, but God was not on board with my plan. His plan involved a process of healing rather than a quick resolution to it.

A short time later, I was standing during the worship time at church, noticing a friend worshiping God a few rows ahead of me. I heard, inside myself, "I can't worship like that; I'm not fixed enough." It occurred to me that I believed that, even as a Christ-follower, my imperfections separated me from God—that I was unacceptable even to Him if I had flaws—or what I would also call "spiritual sickness."

I remembered times when I was physically sick and others didn't want to get close to me because they didn't want to get sick. I remembered times that I felt the same way and distanced myself so I wouldn't get someone else's cold or sickness.

But God was showing me that He didn't need me to get fixed to be in His presence or to worship Him. He showed me that I can worship Him BECAUSE I can be in His presence unfixed, flawed and spiritually sick. I heard Him speak to me, "I will sit with you in your sickness." Not only could I come to Him while having flaws, but He would come to me and stay with me in my sickness.

That was a powerful revelation to me, and it gave me peace as He led me into the next phase of this healing. Since I was now secure in His presence even with flaws, He was able to bring to light even more of my flaws. Each day I was seeing more and more flaws in myself, more and more of things that were wrong with me, but without my newfound security in His acceptance of my sickness and His willingness to sit with me in it, I would have despaired. Instead, while desiring healing and lamenting at my spiritual sickness, I was finding peace in His grace.

In the midst of it all, I found that I was beginning to have an easier time forgiving others and the day-to-day offenses I faced. Because of God's willingness to sit with me in my sickness, my own heart was softening with compassion and understanding that was allowing me to not only forgive, but to sit with others in their spiritual sickness as well.

"'...her sins, which are many, have been forgiven, for she loved much; but he who is forgiven little, loves little.'" (Luke 7:47, NASB)

Kelly, myself and countless others now know an unspeakable freedom, joy and peace of forgiving others that only comes through receiving the ultimate forgiveness: receiving God's unconditional love that He gave when Jesus died the most agonizing death to forgive us our sins and make us right with a perfectly holy God.

CHAPTER 5

TEMPLE CARE

"While donating money, time and one's belongings to the Church is
important, giving your body to the Lord, through adherence to a proper diet
and exercise regime, is one of the most important gifts you can give to
God."
– Matthew Denos

"Dear Friend, I pray that you may enjoy good health and that all may go
well with you, even as your soul is getting along well."
– 3 John 1:2, NLT

Modern-age living has brought many great changes and as many or more great
challenges to our physical wellness. From drive-thrus to microwaves,
remotes to cell phones, internet to ipad, modern convenience and technology have
redefined life as we know it. In this present day, all we have to do for most activities is

press buttons and tap screens. We've literally become paralyzed by modern technology. We sit, we click, we eat, we watch and we sleep. If we choose to, we can live a virtual life through reality shows and facebook, participating in activities in mind only. Some of us don't even know our next door neighbor because we don't even go outside except to get into our air conditioned car. The beautiful noise that was once children playing in the streets has now been silenced by obsessions with video games and ear buds.

The church has gone from being the role model to a "roll" model. Attendees at many churches hear the words of life at the service and then, at the luncheon afterward, they are given sugar and fat packed foods of death.

Remember friends, we are in a literal war for our health. It's a spiritual war of lies and deception. Many food and chemical companies create a false need for junk food. Unhealthy living is made to look glamorous, and healthy living look boring. Just check out a McDonald's or a beer commercial and you can see this. Neither one of these lifestyle examples leads to anything even remotely close to health. If our enemy can steal our physical health, he knows we won't be able to be there to provide for our family, fellowship with believers, or complete the tasks God has given us on this earth.

Nobody really wants to be sick and lazy, do they? I don't see Jesus as an obese couch potato, smoking a cigar, chomping on Doritos with a glass of scotch by His side. The picture we see of Him in the Bible is much different. It's life on the playing field, not in the stands.

God has another life for you to live. It's one that will redefine you from the inside out. There is no way to untie the spiritual, physical and emotional life. God created us as three part beings. We are made in His image. My prayer is that fact alone would be more than enough to spark you to care for your body the very best you can.

God is asking us to take care of all He has given us...

The apostle Paul speaks of disciplining himself in 1 Corinthians 9:24-27 for a crown (prize) that will last forever. He says run in such a way as to get the prize. As he also says, he is not running aimlessly or fighting like a boxer beating the air; he's finding his "wellness" by disciplining himself and having an eternal view of his life. God is asking us to take care of *all* He has given us and to run like the champion He's made us to be, keeping in mind the future here on earth and into eternity. Now and later matters when it comes to temple care.

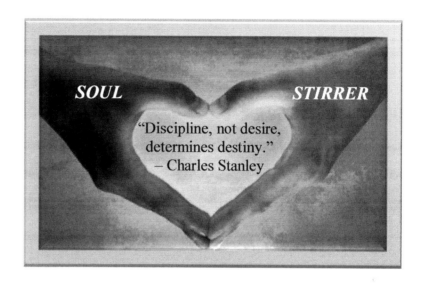

Very often I hear people say "I can't maintain my fitness; I'm just not able to be consistent."

One of the biggest reasons we can't find and/or keep the wellness we desire is that the answers we seek are found in a much deeper place than the body itself. They're found in the soul. The old saying goes, "You can't judge a book by its cover." I tend to believe many times that the opposite is true. The outside is just a reflection of something amiss with the inner person. When I meet someone who is clearly out of shape or starving himself or herself to death on a D-I-E-t, I know there is pain, sorrow or shame hidden below the surface. No one truly wants to look or feel bad. Our identity needs to be in who we are according to what God says in His word, not in anything else. He created us and gave us an amazing intricate physical body. When we understand the importance of our physical health and the connection it has to our spirit, we will have the right motive for caring for our body. God places such an importance on our physical body that He calls it His temple in 1 Corinthians 6:19.

No matter where you are now, you can start again and know what it feels like to be truly alive and well. Even with two near death experiences that resulted from Crohn's disease, I still feel amazing. That has come from the inside out through soul strength. The world says wellness starts from the outside in; God says it starts from the inside and works its way out. I think I'll trust God!

Today I want you to make a life changing decision. Trust God and take Him at His word. Believe that you are truly valuable in His eyes and that He made you and the amazing body He gifted you with for His special purpose. So I say to you, run this race of life on the power of the spirit of the living God, let Him set the pace, and believe that He is with you every step of the way no matter where you are in the race.

Remember this: Your body is the best or worst house you will ever live in.

STRENGTH BUILDERS

1. What value have you typically placed on the physical?

2. What value have you typically placed on the spiritual?

3. What value have you typically placed on the soul?

4. As you consider the inside out approach to temple care, what are the motivation robbers you have to contend with first?

5. What are your goals as it relates to temple care? Write them out and make a commitment.

It's In the Why

In the past three decades I have answered literally thousands of questions on fitness, wellness and lifestyle. Most have asked "What?" and "How?" questions. We do need to ask those, but the most important question to ask ourselves is "Why?" Why am I trying to lose weight? Why do I want to gain muscle? Why am I desiring lifestyle changes?

The reason we so often fail or lose steam quickly is that we really don't know why we're doing what we're doing. The why question is where God will speak to your spirit about motives and where signs of strongholds are revealed. To be honest, the reason most diets don't work is because they're mostly about a short term outward change. Your why needs to come from the inside out, from the soul strength of knowing what God is asking you to do and where He is leading you to go. Make your "why" big enough to create action steps in your life now and in the future. Some examples of big "why" reasons would be "because I don't want to be one of the 1 out of 2 people that will get a life-threatening disease like cancer, heart disease or diabetes, or " I want to be around and healthy enough to play with my kids and grandchildren when I'm older."

There is great blessing and reward for taking the best care of my body that I can. Another very important reason is that I know my family and loved ones learn more from my actions than my words. I want my actions to leave a legacy of wellness and of hope to everyone I know. Even if I live to be 100 there will come a time when I have to give an account of how I took care of what God entrusted to me and those I had influence over. That is a sobering thought I keep at the front of my mind each and every day.

In my early years, my temple was my temptation. I used my body for a weapon instead of a tool in the hands of God. Because of my self-promotion, I was really scoring points for the enemy. I filled myself with the toxins of people-worship and success. Truthfully, I built a wall of muscle around a broken soul. I found out the hard way that if your only reason to "better" yourself is external, and maybe how you look to others, then you are building a glass house that will eventually shatter from the rocks that comparison will throw at it. Fortunately, God is a God of grace, and through soul strength Jesus changed my mind and heart, but not without some heavenly hard knocks. I was on a diet of eating my own words and on a training program lifting the much too heavy weights of shame and regret. God graciously helped me get out of my own way and led me back to a place where I could see myself through His eyes and a place where I was teachable and able to be used by Him in ways I could never imagine.

STRENGTH BUILDERS

1. List your "Why" questions here.

2. Now, take some time to consider and answer your "Why" questions.

3. Has your temple been your area of temptation? Explain.

4. Have you put walls up to guard your hurts and brokenness? What, if any, is the hesitancy in having those walls removed?

Don'ts and can'ts are two huge boulders that block wellness success.

They must be removed or you will remain exactly where you are today.

We can all list a million reasons why we don't have the time to exercise or eat right. The two I hear most often are, "I don't have the time to work out" and "It costs too much to eat right." Here is the truth: If you don't have time to exercise now, you *will* have time for disease later. If you think eating well is too expensive, then you'll end up with the cost of treating disease. There is a universal law to which we all must answer: play now and pay later, or pay now and play later. Financial expert Dave Ramsey has a saying that I think hits it right on the head. Although he uses it when talking about finances, it can definitely be used when talking about health and the body. It goes like this: "Live like no one else so that later you can live like no one else." In other words, you need to think about and plan for the future and take action, now. If you don't, you won't have one.

I know from my own life, and from training and counseling thousands of people over the years, that God will make you more than able to get past the past, beyond the excuses, and overcome what I call negative verbal forecasting. Doing this will put you in the starting blocks for a brand new life. Simple education in mind, body and spirit can lengthen and even save your life. Hosea 4:6 says, "My people are destroyed from lack of knowledge." The context of this passage is referring to Israel and the failure of priests, but in the New Testament, God calls Christians priests. (1 Peter 2:5) We need head and heart knowledge to gain wellness and victory in the physical.

The very first thing I want you to do is remove "I can't" and "I don't" from your vocabulary. We do more damage to our future by these words than just about anything else. Saying it automatically disqualifies you from even beginning to better yourself. Start reciting "I am willing, and God is able." Even if you improve 1% a day, in three months you'll be 90% better. Anyone can do 1% a day.

STRENGTH BUILDERS

1. What are some of the reasons you have used or are using that prevent you from taking steps to change?

2. What are some ways you plan to get more educated in this area? (Hosea 4:6)

Temple Foundations

For any house (or temple) to stand sturdy throughout the years it needs a strong foundation. The fuel you put in your body *is* the foundation on which it stands or falls. You can do all the exercise you want, but if you don't fuel your body with real living foods you won't feel or look your best.

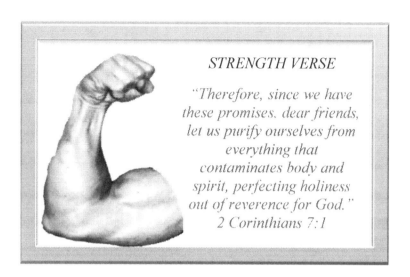

STRENGTH VERSE

"Therefore, since we have these promises, dear friends, let us purify ourselves from everything that contaminates body and spirit, perfecting holiness out of reverence for God."
2 Corinthians 7:1

I want to give you something to pin on your mind and your heart and to stick on your refrigerator that will be a great motivator for fueling your body correctly. You are eating for three: God, you and your loved ones. Honor God by taking care of His property (your body), be at peak performance to do all that He's called you to do, and be there for the long haul for your loved ones. They need you.

For detailed guidance and consideration on nutrition and exercise, please go to Appendix B in the back of this book, beginning on page 149.

Becoming a "Dangerously" Great Temple for God

Dangerous is a good thing here because you will be a temple warrior who not only is winning the war against the enemy of the body but is leading others on to victory as well. As you understand the value God has placed on your life, you will see how important it is to Him and to you to practice temple care daily. This is not a 90 day challenge, although something like that is very helpful for a jump start. This is a mindset and lifestyle of the seeds of greatness God has grown in you. The soul strength life needs to be engrained in your DNA. When you know who you are in Christ, you hear His voice clearly, you act by the power of the spirit, not the flesh, and you lead others to wholeness in spirit, mind and body. You can have a dangerously well-tuned mind and body that is a walking billboard for God's design for life.

There is one last piece to this puzzle. To maintain greatness in our temple, we need to have a like-minded set of inner circle relationships, a safe place to share any struggles and a place of strength and encouragement. A well armored temple army is not easily defeated! Look for those who are like-minded and want to reach their full potential for God. I would not have made such gains if I didn't have great workout and accountability partners cheering me on and pushing me beyond my limits. Going it alone makes it easier to get discouraged or fail.

Remember, we are all a work in progress, so if it took you 20-30 years to get to where you are physically, don't expect to get where you need to go in two to three weeks. Start a new mindset about food and exercise. Food is a luxury and the body is a gift. Food is fuel to nourish us and keep us on the planet longer to accomplish God's purposes. Our body carries our spirit and it needs to be at peak performance to not only meet the demands of daily life, but to accomplish God's work here on earth. We only have a certain amount of time here. We can spend it or invest it, but we can never get it

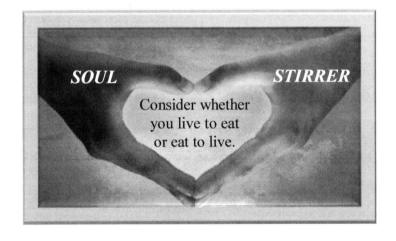

SOUL **STIRRER**

Consider whether you live to eat or eat to live.

back. Consider it a privilege to take care of God's masterpiece.

Also, be mindful as you journey to health and wholeness. Don't ever forget that you have someone who wants to take you out. The evil one is a mind-manipulating liar. He will mess with your thinking and your body if you let him. Your enemy wants you to believe he has control over you and is all powerful. He is not! If he was, I wouldn't be here today.

I can honestly say that I love who I am today. This doesn't come from ego, but from my Creator who made me. For many years people have come to see me speak because they've seen me on television, and because of my physique, but God has so transformed my life with soul strength that there is now what I call a bait and switch that happens. I surrender to His will and message so they will not only hear the words the Lord wants for their hearts but are hopefully directed to a path that puts Jesus first in their lives. My mission is making Him known in my voice, soul and body.

God has also shown me that along my journey I needed mentors and accountability in my life to lift me up and inspire me to be the best I can be. Frank Zane and Jack LaLanne were both heroes to me. I looked up to them because they were at the top of their game, they had confidence in who they were, and I also wanted to look just like them. Deep honest friendships are so important to me. My "inner circle" of close friends is always there to listen and love on me as I share my deepest hurts. They also share in my excitement when I tell them a dream or goal God has laid on my heart. I know that I can call them day or night, and if I have a need, they will do whatever they need to so that need will be met. In short, it's a family. God also gave me a spiritual mentor and father-in-the-faith, Paul Bersche. He has given me sound biblical counsel and calls me to the carpet when necessary.

With the help of God, mentors and accountability partners, no matter what shape your temple is currently in, you can make the choice to clean the slate and start again. Each morning God's mercies are new, so start your day off by asking Him to be your training partner for spirit, soul and body, and you will be

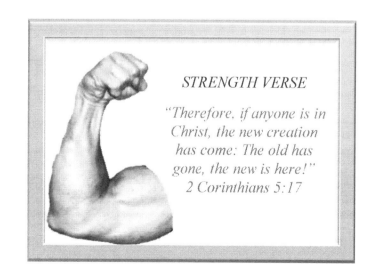

STRENGTH VERSE

"Therefore, if anyone is in Christ, the new creation has come: The old has gone, the new is here!"
2 Corinthians 5:17

astounded at what He will do and who He'll bring to you on this incredible journey called life. Your return for this investment is eternal.

STRENGTH BUILDERS

1. Besides the accountability partner you are seeking out, who else will be part of your network of support as you endeavor to change?

2. Are you currently being coached/ led/ mentored by someone that would be willing to support the changes you are making through this study? Seek someone out if not. List some names of potential mentors.

3. What are the potential benefits you will reap by allowing others to be part of this journey with you?

Attitude—The Key That Turns Every Lock*

It's all about health, fitness and lifestyle. In this attitude, I have found a key that turns every lock, enhances every situation in my life and puts me on the best possible path to negotiate life. It's far more than muscles and aerobic capacity and body fat percentages.

It's about wanting the very best health for yourself and the one and only vehicle that will carry you through your life. The good habits, self-discipline and emotional balance required to achieve glowing health will permeate every facet of a person's life.

As I worked my way from a hospital bed to a Brooklyn gym to championship stages to a fitness career in Detroit, I learned over and over, ever more deeply, that I couldn't have a healthy and fit body unless I had a healthy and fit life. So for me, it's no small message when I say that it's about health, fitness and lifestyle. Now that message is the theme of my syndicated television program by the same name: "Peter's Principles".

The lesson that I have continued to learn, that I can still trace back to that turning point at the Verazzano Narrows Bridge, is that health and fitness serve not just my body, but also my whole self, my whole soul. Sure, fitness makes the body good to look at; it also gives it the best possible chance to avoid and fight disease. But the key that turns every lock

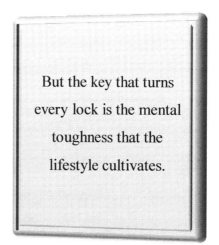

But the key that turns every lock is the mental toughness that the lifestyle cultivates.

is the mental toughness that the lifestyle cultivates. I'm not talking about tough like Clint Eastwood or Xena. I'm talking about the toughness you need to make the right decision at the dinner table, every time you choose between the TV and a workout, *every* time you choose to do the right thing. That toughness starts to spill over into other aspects of your life, like deciding not to retaliate against some road-raged driver to deciding to be a positive influence instead of a complainer. It builds on itself, and it pays off tenfold during those moments of truth—during crisis. It ensures that not only is the body in the best possible shape to respond, but so is the mind.

Consistent healthy living is like making investments in a mental fortitude account.

A fit attitude and mental toughness help us to be resilient to those unavoidable setbacks we all experience. Setbacks are a part of progress, and I've had my share. Some have been recent; some I recall vividly from early in my career.

I remember being sick, somewhere around age 20. I was at the family apartment—the nest I often returned to when things weren't right. I remember being upstairs, and a friend had stopped by for a visit. I developed cramps that were so bad I thought I'd need an ambulance. My mother wanted me to go to the corner store to get something for dinner, and there I sat with that old terror and denial descending on me all over again.

In a panic, I asked myself: "How could this be happening?" I had already won a major teenage bodybuilding championship. I thought I "had my health back." You know, *for good*. I had been feeling great. And there I was, terrified all over again that I couldn't hold my bowels long enough to get to the corner and back. Was I so fragile that even after all that work I could suddenly, without warning, fall apart? I had to really take an honest look at my habits and lifestyle, and there were some contributing factors.

The bottom line was that I had been taking my health for granted again—not really watching what I ate, thinking that if a body looks great on the outside everything must be great on the inside. Common (expensive) mistake. Meanwhile, I was also breaking up with a girlfriend, and just to spice it up a little, a car I liked a lot had just been stolen—and now I was having a relapse. The lesson? Taking my health for granted is a temptation I can't afford. It can cost me everything.

It's tough to toe the line at that age; cockiness is just part of growing up, part of finding one's independence from the family, I guess. Unfortunately for me, it was far more of a luxury than I could afford, when it came to my health. It was a hard time, but I got back on my feet fast.

Around that time a song called "Eye of the Tiger" was getting a lot of airtime. The lyrics talked about how quickly we can change, how easy it is to trade passion for glory—to focus on the rewards of doing the right thing, forgetting about the right thing itself. (The name of the band was Survivor, to add a poetic touch.) It also talked about getting back on your feet and getting back out there after a fall. I really took that message to heart as a young man trying to keep his priorities straight, and that song meant a great deal to me for many years. Much of my life so far had been devoted to learning that lesson. I like to think that by now I've learned it fairly well.

...crises will happen regardless of who we are and what we want,

and we have to be prepared to face them head-on.

Crohn's was always a great reminder. I've had four major setbacks in 20 years; three were in the first 10 years, and only one in the last 10. Each time, I thought I had "arrived"—that the disease was in the permanent remission. And each time nature reminded me that life is short, the path is tricky and there are no guarantees. I gradually learned not to take things for granted. And to be mentally prepared for anything—as the saying goes, "hope for the best, but prepare for the worst." Thankfully, I learned a little bit more from that mistake every time. Because of the Crohn's, I am much less able to wander off the straight and narrow because the repercussions are so costly.

Another particularly ill-timed "curve ball" took place 13 days before I got on a plane to Belize to win the biggest title I'd competed for so far, at that time. It seemingly came out of nowhere—BOOM—like somebody cut me off at the knees. This time I was heavily into training, eating exactly the right foods—and still here comes the Crohn's. Unbelievable! I remember looking at myself in the mirror, slapping myself in the face saying: "There's no way you can get sick." Guess again. I calmed down, but I was not in the best health when I won that competition. The lesson was that crises will happen regardless of who we are and what we want, and we have to be prepared to face them head-on.

...the investment I had been making for years in my body and mind paid off, and I weathered the storm.

This is why I talk about mistakes, obstacles and crises. You can correct mistakes in your life. You can fight obstacles and manage crises, but you can't prevent them. Taking care of yourself, developing the most positive mental outlook and the healthiest lifestyle possible is *no guarantee* that you won't be hit by a debilitating disease or some other crisis. Only God knows that. You could get hit by a bus tomorrow. But I can guarantee you that the right lifestyle and attitude will help you prevent the predictable ones, and sometimes vastly improve the outcome of the unavoidable ones. At the very least, a healthy mental attitude will help counteract denial and other destructive responses to a crisis.

I had read the recipe for good living, and I was following instructions, and still I got hit again. But the investment I had been making for years in my body and mind paid off, and I weathered the storm.

Sometimes the biggest risk we deal with during a setback or a crisis is the temptation to sink into self-pity. That song I referred to earlier also talked about having a fire inside, a burning desire to make it. I developed that fire because I was blessed with adversity and because I followed through on the commitment I made to get well. Being sick gave me tremendous desire to be well. It motivated me to learn how the body works, how to use it and what to put in it. I work out. I eat well. I have confidence. And because I look good, I have even more confidence. It's a total package: priorities, values, self-love, love for others, health, fitness—and they all feed on each other, one piece supporting another. And that's the whole point.

My most important message is this: There are many components to that total package, but nobody can have the *whole package* unless fitness is part of the picture. *Anybody* can find that fire within themselves and become that whole package. You just start by doing the best you can, one day at a time, for the body you're going to have to live in 24 hours a day, cradle to grave. That commitment never ends, no matter how fit you get. (*Nielsen)

STRENGTH BUILDERS

1. What are some areas you need to change your attitude in to make it more "fit" for your future goals?

2. Reflect and write about some of the obstacles, challenges and crises you have faced so far in this life? What have been the consequences? What have been the lessons learned?

3. If you were able to go back in time and have a "do over", what attitude changes would you make that could have changed the outcome?

4. Write out an attitude commitment statement for your "temple goals".

Every day we get a present called today. We are given 86,400 precious seconds. Whether they are spent or invested, when the day ends and the clock strikes twelve, they are gone, and you can never get them back.

Are you maximizing

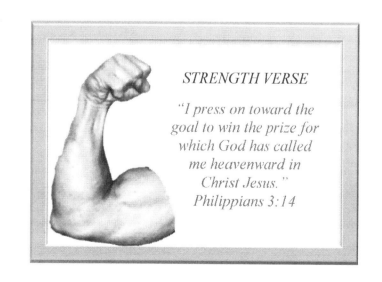

STRENGTH VERSE

"I press on toward the goal to win the prize for which God has called me heavenward in Christ Jesus."
Philippians 3:14

and investing your gift of today? If not, what changes need to take place for you to do this?

Be an investor of this gift of today and be an investor in the gift of *His* temple and you will reap great rewards in this life and the next.

"Every good and perfect gift is from above, coming down from the father
of the heavenly lights, who does not change like shifting shadows."

– James 1:17

CHAPTER 6

LOVE

"Three things will last forever—faith, hope, and love—and the greatest
of these is love."
– 1 Corinthians 13:13, NLT

F riends, if there is a glue that holds each chapter of this book and my entire life
together, it's love. You simply cannot have soul strength or a fulfilled,
meaningful life without it. In every area of my life, no matter what I say or do, I strive to
have the main ingredient be love—not the love I produce, but the love God has produced
in me.

"Three things will last forever—faith, hope, and love—and the greatest of these is
love." (1 Corinthians 13:13, NLT)

Of all the words I can think of, love is the most overused, perverted and under
practiced. It is often described as a feeling, something we fall in and out of, and is very
often confused with lust.

If I were to ask you, "how's your love life?" where would your mind go? Our minds have been programmed by the world to go straight to the physical or romantic love, and even to lustful thoughts. What about God? What about the Creator of love? What about your relationship with the One who *is* love? What would it be like if the immediate thought that penetrated your mind when asked that question was your love relationship with your Creator? It's my prayer that by the end of this chapter your answer to the question will be this: "God *is* my love life, and my love life is amazing!"

Look at the world around us and how its "love" influence has molded generations. Think for a moment about how the power of music/song has influenced and redefined our definition of love. What "love" message has the most

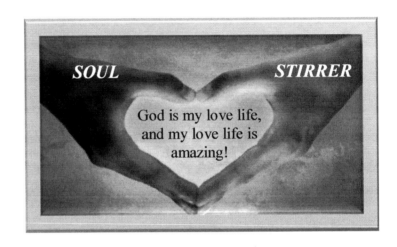

popular love songs over the past fifty years given us about true love? It's confusing at best. Frankie Lymon and the Teenagers asked, "why do fools fall in love?", the Beatles said, "love is all you need", Elvin Bishop "fooled around and fell in love", Queen called it "a crazy little thing", Robert Palmer's diagnosis was, "you might as well face it you're addicted to it", Phil Collins had a "groovy kind of love", J Geils just said "it stinks", Madonna justified her love, Tina Turner asked, "what's love got to do with it?", and concluded that it was "just a second hand emotion." Foreigner, at least said, "I want to know what love is." Now remember these were all number one hits throughout the years that infiltrated and impacted hearts and minds about what love was all about. The question we need to ask is, "What did they say about real love?" The answer: nothing! There is no defined or lasting meaning in them.

Television wasn't exactly a GPS to real love either. The Love Boat, Everybody Loves Raymond, I Love Lucy, The Love Connection. Think about how much influence our upbringing, friends, TV, radio and all of media have on our understanding of love. It's staggering to think of everything our minds have taken in over the years. No wonder we've had a hard time understanding what defines real love and how to apply it in our lives. Human kind's definition of love always programs us to fail because it's usually based on feelings and circumstances.

Human kind's definition of love always programs us to fail

because it's usually based on feelings and circumstances.

Lust, Lies and Lowering the Bar

For generations now, the standard of love has fallen far from what God originally intended. What was once pornography was turned into "free love." One study confirmed that "children are exposed to more violence, sexuality, harsh language, and drug use in G, PG, and PG-13 movies these days than they were just a few years ago." (MPAA rating system) Movie content that was once Rated X and Rated R is now creeping into our own and our children's lives through PG and PG-13 ratings.

What was once a sacred institution, marriage, got reduced to the "safer" version of shacking up, where just in case everything doesn't go as planned, the back door to "freedom" is left unlocked and slightly ajar. Our love has become a contract signed in pencil that we've allowed ourselves to re-write as conditions or our feelings change. The gradual cheapening of this glorious gift from God has left the world in a confused mess. What are the glorious results of making our own master plan to redefine love? More divorce, more disease, moral decay and a very desensitized society. The canvas God uses to paint His love masterpiece is our heart, but to do that, He must first clean off the messy fingerprints that have been left there by our past, the influence of the world and our own sin nature.

STRENGTH BUILDER

1. How has your definition of love been influenced by media?

Searching for Love in All the Wrong Places

Lust (which has become the standard) and love, are mutually exclusive. We keep searching for this beautiful treasure of love from the outside in. The aesthetics of humans and things command the attention of our eyes, filling us temporarily with the thrill of now, but leaving us lacking in the fulfillment of the long term. God unveils the truth about this kind of "love" in 1 John 2:16 (NLT): "For the world offers only a craving for physical pleasure, a craving for everything we see, and pride in our achievements and possessions. These are not from the Father, but are from this world."

Ponder for a moment the stark contrast between love and lust. Lust demands; love gives. Lust honors self; love is selfless. Lust leads to disappointment; love leads to God. God is love and love is the fulfillment of everything good! When it comes to love, we've been given a precious gift of choice. We can choose His love or the world's dysfunctional version of love. There was a time I would have chosen the world's version of love because it seemed so satisfying to me. I have come to learn that no matter how good it tastes, how good it smells, how good it looks, if it doesn't match up with God's definition of love, it can't fulfill the deepest longings of our hearts.

The true you (which is your spirit) cannot be satisfied with the lust of the flesh. In my life, the enemy of my soul observed my "flesh" tendencies and, at just the right time, put sparkly objects like women, cars and substances directly in my path. He deceived me into thinking they could satisfy the deepest longings of my heart. This deception put me on an endless and relentless quest to fill this love gap with everything this world could offer. But you know what? It was *never* enough. We all have holes, and when we try to fill them with people, things and substances, we will still leak. They can't stop the hunger God placed in us that only He can satisfy. His love alone will cement those holes shut and stop the leaks. When He covers the leaks, then we can be filled and whole. The problem most of us have is that we want to mix some of God's love with some of the world's, and it's a volatile combination. God will, by His gift of free will, let you choose who/what you will serve and allow to fill you, but He won't let you choose to serve Him *and* His enemy's false love.

That's why my life was in such torment. I was trying to serve two masters. The true satisfaction and fulfillment that I now know came only when I stopped pursuing the things of this world as my definition of love. The devil offers us counterfeits for God's love on every corner—objects, people, success and money are all appealing "lovers" that can capture our hearts and draw us away from God's perfect love with a short term satisfaction. The world around us has eroticized the sacred gift of intimacy and prompts us to paint pictures of sex on the screen of our minds and call it love. God created physical as well as all other forms of intimacy. It's a pure gift that comes

> "For God so loved the world that he gave his one and only Son, so that whoever believes in him shall not perish but have eternal life."
> – John 3:16

from Him and is made to glorify His name. The deepest form of intimacy (into-me-you-see) should be with our Creator. Searching for love in all the wrong places will eventually lead us down a path to emptiness and disappointment every time.

Recently someone asked me what God's definition of love was and how it looks in action. My immediate answer was, *JESUS!* John 3:16 popped into my mind right away: "For God so loved the world that he gave his one and only Son, that whoever believes in him shall not perish but have eternal life." God sent love in a person; it's not a man-made formula. Love defined everything Jesus was and everything He did. He was and is Love! Real love isn't a feeling we get from an emotional experience, or physical pleasure, it's Jesus Himself! Sacrificial, selfless, unconditional love! When we ask Him to be lord and master of our lives, He comes in and plants soul strength seeds in us so we will be able to hear His voice, have the power of His spirit and model His love.

STRENGTH BUILDERS

1. Have you confused lust with love in your past? How?

2. Do you find it difficult to embrace God's perfect definition of love? If so, why?

When Love Hurts

Some of those messy fingerprints on our hearts were left there by mom or dad. We all have a model of love that was built for us from a young age, most likely by our parents. As a child, love may have been spelled out to you (as it was in my life) p.a.i.n. or f.e.a.r.

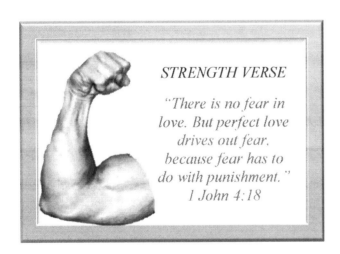

STRENGTH VERSE

"There is no fear in love. But perfect love drives out fear, because fear has to do with punishment."
1 John 4:18

In our home, the picture of what God considers love was truly distorted, although, at the time it was all I knew. Anxiety, lack of trust and fear were normal to me. When sin and selfish love master lives, there is no low to which we can't fall. Unfortunately, what I (and many of you) went through as a child is not that uncommon.

Many times I've pondered the thought of how different it would have been for our family if my dad had had soul strength and had been able to hear, receive and act on God's model of true love.

Fortunately, God will use any circumstance to draw us to Him, and that's exactly what He wants to do in your life. As Charles Stanley says, "He will move heaven and earth to show you His will." Sometimes it feels like hell is what's moving, but don't ever forget God is *always* in control, *always* interested in all you are going through (even the smallest detail), and His love will *never* fail you, ever!

First John 4:18 says, "There is no fear in love. But perfect love drives out fear, because fear has to do with punishment." God's perfect love gave me freedom from the fear and pain that defined my childhood.

STRENGTH BUILDER

1. Write out the definition of love that you understood from your family of origin.

Self Love and Boundaries

Codependency is described as, "persons [who] are drawn to relationships in which they must take care of the emotional needs of others in a way that is harmful to their own spiritual and emotional health." (Sledge) Codependency masquerades as love in many marriages and relationships. Make no mistake, love is not tolerance or "anything goes." Love tells the truth, stands up for what is right and does not condone sinful behavior. Peace at all cost is not what love is all about. You shouldn't be a doormat remaining in potentially dangerous situations where someone is harming you. Abuse is not a part of real love.

Boundaries are necessary in proper self-love. Allowing abusive behavior and an absence of boundaries will distort the truth of love that God wants you to have. You have options and you were created to be loved properly. You are a creation and treasure of God himself! Reaching out for help is power. Prayer is power. Believing is power. God will bring safe people into your life that can give you His healing love and help bring you out of your current situation if there is codependency.

Proper self love is also based on our identity. Who we believe we are determines how we will act and react to situations in our lives. If we aren't convinced of our deep value, we will have a tendency to look for codependent relationships because we think we can get our worth in people and what they think of us. If we are convinced of the value that God says we have, and we know that God, by His love, created us and we mattered so much to Him that He sacrificed His only son so we didn't have to pay the penalty for our sins, then we will live life a completely different way—a way that honors God and honors self.

Seeing ourselves through His eyes will give us the desire to take care of our body, mind and spirit, and remove ourselves from harmful, abusive situations. When we see the lengths God went through to create us and the world that He gave us to enjoy, we can't help but love His creation, of which we are His crowning jewel. We are the only creature made in His image.

*His sacrificial death gave us life and forgiveness of all of our sins —
past, present and future.*

Receiving and giving are both a part of God's plan for our love life. Sometimes we find it very difficult to receive a gift from someone and not feel obligated to give something back. This goes to a much deeper level when it concerns receiving the forgiving love of God. We often feel completely unworthy and undeserving, but by the cross Christ bore on our behalf, we are worthy. His sacrificial death gave us life and forgiveness of *all* of our sins—past, present and future. His love doesn't ask for pay backs or "I owe you" contracts. His only "ask" of you is that you trust His love and receive His forgiveness. Our obedience, behavior and giving back to God results from us being changed by His perfect love by first making a home in our heart. We become conduits for that love as we "witness" for Christ by extending His love to others and telling them about Him.

We actually witness about things all the time and don't even realize it. You tell people about that awesome movie you just saw or the great new song that just came out, and that's fine, but think about a witness that can actually change a life for eternity. When Jesus and His love live in you, you can't help but tell people about what He has done for you and how He radically changed your life.

So, you're saying:

> *Peter, my daily life isn't even close to being filled with love right now. I am divorced, have an abusive background, I'm lonely, and judgment from others is what I've been receiving daily. I'm not feeling God's love in my heart at all.*

Please don't feel all alone in this. Many of us have endured hardships, abuse and loneliness in short or long seasons. This resonates deeply within my heart because of the trials in my own life, and I don't take lightly anyone who tells me they are struggling in their life. I've been there and have seen the darkest days that seemed like they would never go away. That is why I am so passionate about the love of God. That amazing, unconditional love completely changed my life from the inside out. I promise you, God is pursuing you right now and is very aware of your situation. He loves you! It may seem impossible for you to love or be loved right now, but don't let that steal your hope.

I want you to rethink possible, and, by the power of soul strength, expand your boundaries of *can*. With God, you can see on the other side of too far, too hard, or impossible. Being filled with God's love, I see impossible in a brand new way. I see it as *I'm possible!* Although hard

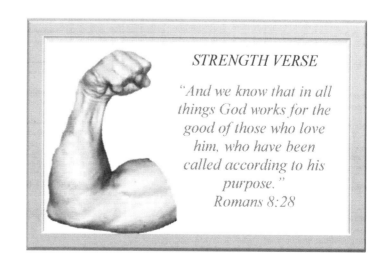

STRENGTH VERSE

"And we know that in all things God works for the good of those who love him, who have been called according to his purpose."
Romans 8:28

117

to understand during my trials, God was making me more like His son, Jesus. He was right there with me in the midst of my pain making the impossible possible! The perfect love of a father loves, molds, disciplines, and at times, lets growth come about by allowing struggles to build strength and Christ-like character. It was actually the hurts and heartaches in my life that have given me the ability to honestly say to people who are going through the same thing, "I understand", and mean it. I wouldn't be able to give guidance and show them a testimony of living hope otherwise.

Romans 8:28 says, "And we know that in all things God works for the good of those who love him, who have been called according to his purpose."

STRENGTH BUILDERS

1. Now that you have the hope of good coming from bad situations and a new perspective to consider, write about a time that comes to mind where you can now clearly see something good coming from a situation that seemed impossible.

2. Is there a current situation that you need to stand in faith that God is going to bring good? Share that with a trusted friend and have them pray with you specifically about it.

I am living proof that God's love is perfect, patient and *very* real. I'm often reminded of a passage that has always given me hope and a right perspective on God's love during the periods of struggle and the times when love seemed absent. It's a solid reminder that when I cry out to Him, His love is present and His help is on the way. It's found in

Matthew chapter 7, verse 11: "So if you sinful people know how to give good gifts to your children, how much more will your heavenly father give good gifts to those who ask him." My dad did some very sinful things to my mom, me and our family, but even he had the capacity to, at times, give good gifts.

Experience may damage, but God's love restores and will fill all the lack with abundance. He has given me gifts of His love beyond anything I could imagine! He doesn't ask for paybacks either. As I have received that love from my perfect Heavenly Father, I joyfully and willing give everything I am to Him each day of my life—even an imperfect earthly daddy like me. I know God's love flows through me and I love to shower my two beautiful daughters with it as much as I possibly can.

If your life experience has, or is, lacking in love from your parents, family or relationships, please don't lose hope. God will (just like He did in my life) reparent, reposition and also replenish the love you lost or are lacking. His love gives you just what you need to overcome and prosper in Him. In fact, He's promised in His Word, much more than you could ever imagine. Ephesians 3:20-21 says, "Now to him who is able to do immeasurably more than all we ask or imagine, according to his power that is at work within us, to him be glory in the church and in Christ Jesus throughout all generations, for ever and ever! Amen."

Isolation almost cost me everything...

Another way God expresses His love is through people. I cannot stress enough how healthy relationships and a community of believers have brought healing to me and drawn me closer to God in ways I could never have imagined. There is nothing weak about getting help, seeking advice and confessing your struggles to those who are safe and trustworthy. Isolation almost cost me everything at one point in my life. If you stay isolated from people, chances are you will want to hide from God as well. If you stay on your own little island of pain, shame or pity, you will never have the comfort and healing God wants you to have. Unity expressed in love has great power.

"Do not fear" is said again and again in God's Word for a reason. If the devil can get you to fear, he's got you in his trap. Don't be afraid to ask God to bring healthy people into your life that will come alongside you and love you without judgment. I'm always concerned when I talk to someone that says, "I can handle this." That self-power and isolation will always end in disappointment and failure. We *all* need community, we *all* need mentoring, and we *all* need the help of others. God designed us for relationship. When we first have a relationship with Him, we will know what real love looks like, then we can choose relationships with people that reflect His love. That reflection needs to be *very* evident especially when it comes to choosing relationships that could potentially lead to marriage. It is a must that you choose someone who is on the same page with you spiritually. Ladies, make sure the man you want to marry is a man after God's own heart and that his life clearly reflects God's love and purity. Men, find a woman (as Max Lucado says) whose heart is so hidden in God that a man has to seek Him just to find her. Marriage is God made, God given and needs to be God honoring. It is a covenant, not a contract; a commitment, not a convenience. Ask God for soul strength to choose the right mate, and also by His love living in you, to become the right mate. And as I mentioned earlier about those "holes" we have. Fill them with God first, and then you won't be looking for someone to complete you, but someone to complement you, because you've already been completed in Christ and His fullness of love.

STRENGTH BUILDERS

1. Share a time someone loved you with a love that you knew was beyond human experience. How did it impact you?

2. Pray and ask God to love others through you this week and document it in a journal.

To truly give and receive love in any relationship, we must take off any "mask" we may be wearing. We feel we need to hide our "blemishes" and imperfections to be accepted, so we wear different masks at different times to keep them hidden. We do this at parties, in friendships, families, and yes, even before God. Being honest and open, first with God, and also with people will allow both the giving and receiving of love to flow freely, and the healing of the heart to begin. There is true freedom and a much greater ability to receive love when we take our mask off. Blemishes and imperfections are a reality of our lives this side of heaven. Read this story below. It describes the pain, shame and loneliness of someone living life wearing a mask.

"The Mask"*

Don't be fooled by me.

Don't be fooled by the face I wear;

for I wear a mask—a thousand masks,

masks that I'm afraid to take off,

and none of them are really me.

Pretending is an art that's second nature to me,

but don't be fooled.

I give you the impression that I'm secure,

that all is sunny and unruffled with me, within as well as without.

Confidence is my name and coolness is my game.

I am in command. I need no one.

But don't believe me—please.

My surface may seem smooth but my surface is my mask—

my ever-changing and ever-concealing mask.

Beneath dwells the real me in confusion, in fear, in aloneness.

But I hide this. I don't want anybody to know it.

I panic at the thought of my fear and weakness being exposed.

That's why I frantically create a mask to hide behind,

a nonchalant, sophisticated facade—to help me pretend,

to shield me.

Acceptance, followed by love is what I need.

It is one thing that will assure me that I'm really worth something.

But I don't tell you this. I don't dare. I'm afraid to.

I'm afraid that you'll think less of me,

that you'll laugh, and your laugh would kill me.

My life becomes a front.

I idly chatter to you in the suave tones of surface talk.

I tell you everything that's really nothing,

and nothing of what's everything.

So when I'm going through my routine,

do not be fooled by what I'm saying.

Please listen carefully and try to hear what I'm not saying,

what I'd like to be able to say, but what I'm afraid to say.

I dislike the superficial game I'm playing—

the superficial, phony game.

I'd really like to be genuine and spontaneous and me.

But that fear—that wall of fear—it stops me every time.

My survival depends on breaking through that wall.

It depends on me…fighting my fear,

shedding my mask and showing myself to you.

But I am scared.

I'm afraid that deep down I'm nothing—that I'm just no good,

and that you'll see this and reject me.

So, I play my game, my desperate, pretending game,

with a facade of assurance without,

and a trembling child within,

and so begins the parade of masks.

*Adapted from the original poem, "Please Hear What I'm Not Saying" by Charles C. Finn

Does this resemble what you're going through? Can you relate to this in any way? If so, then you need this truth:

Masks are a prison sentence that can last a lifetime if we let them. You'll never fully experience soul strength until you can take the mask off. God knows the real you, and He wants the whole you, blemishes and all. He knows you inside and out. Psalm 139 says He knows all our ways, there is nowhere we can flee from His presence and that He knit us together in our mother's womb. He knows us! His love and the love of His people come pouring in as we offer ourselves and our wounds openly and honestly. He loves you exactly as you are and His amazing plan for you is to be where you will experience life and love abundantly. Don't be afraid to take that mask off. Fear is the cancer to your experiencing real love. I often say that life is found in the dance between your deepest desire to love and your deepest fear.

STRENGTH BUILDERS

1. Are you being challenged by this information to take off a mask? In order to do so, you need to believe there are benefits to doing so. Write out the benefits you will experience if you take off your mask.

The Language of Love

God speaks His love to us in many different "languages." Did you know you have a love language? This is a particular "language" where you can hear God's voice and feel His presence strongest. For some, it's music/song. You might feel His presence so strongly in a lyric or melody that it will stop you in your tracks, or even bring you to your knees in praise as if He's right in front of you. For others it may be corporate worship. It may be out in the beautiful nature that He created looking at a magnificent sunset, feeling the warm breeze of spring, or watching the effortless glide of a bird in the sky and experiencing His undeniable presence.

2. So, what is your love language? In what ways do you experience God's presence the strongest?

Whatever it may be, I suggest you purposefully make time to pursue Him through that. Whether it be corporate worship, getting alone in prayer, enjoying praise music, basking in the beauty of the outdoors, or whatever else reveals God to your heart, go there and do that. I guarantee, you will enjoy the life-changing power of His undeniable voice, His language of love, spoken out loud to your spirit.

As you receive the perfect, unconditional and saving love of Jesus into your heart, you will start to live out the example of real love we see in 1 Corinthians 13:4-7. Ask God to fill you to the full with His love and give you the soul strength to love just like Him. I want you to read this passage from 1 Corinthians 13 out loud and fill your name in each blank.

_____ is patient, _____ is kind,

_____ does not envy, _____ does not boast,

_____ is not proud, _____ is not rude,

_____ is not self-seeking, _____ is not easily angered,

_____ keeps no record of wrongs,

_____ does not delight in evil, but rejoices with the truth.

_____ always protects, always trusts, always hopes, always perseveres.

In this fallen world, we will never be perfect, but His perfect love is taking us on a journey heavenward in His perfection.

I will leave you with these final truths: Love does not stink, and love is not a second hand emotion. And, I am going to answer the "I want to know what love is" question that Foreigner posed almost thirty years ago, but in order to do so there needs to be a correction. Love is not a *what*; it's a *who*.

It's *JESUS!*

So, I will ask again. How's your love life?

My prayer is that *His* love rule and reign in your heart and *His* truth be lived out in your life each and every day.

CHAPTER 7

FINISHING STRONG

"One of the most powerful motivators in life is your purpose."
– P. N. N.

"However, I consider my life worth nothing to me; my only aim is to finish
the race and complete the task the Lord Jesus has given me—the task of
testifying to the good news of God's grace."
– Acts 20:24

This is my personal soul strength verse. It's a reminder to my spirit of the true purpose of my earthly life.

A friend recently asked me, if it were possible to hear the words of my eulogy at my own funeral, what I would like to hear. I replied with this:

I never saw the man without a smile. If I didn't know him better I would think it was all an act. Whenever he opened his mouth, words of God's love, peace and hope flowed out. No matter what happened in his life, he saw the good in it and the lesson to be learned. He helped others find their passion in life and finish the race strong. Even though he was programmed to fail because of his abusive childhood, God gave him his hope back. He was never ever afraid to talk about his love affair with Jesus.

So, if someone were to ask you the same question, what would your answer be? If you were to die tonight, what kind of picture of your life would be portrayed in the words said by those who knew you best? It's a sobering question, I know, but one we all need to ask ourselves.

We've all heard the stock answers at countless funerals. Common phrases are, "He was a proud man," or "He was a hard worker," or even (cringe) "He could party with the best of them."

Be honest, how are you finishing life? Limping? Careless? Angry? Are you on auto-pilot? Are you just hoping for the best?

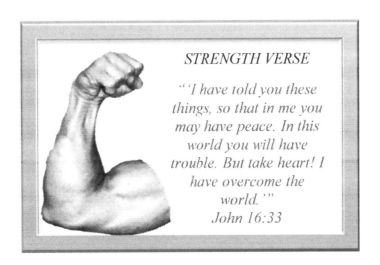

STRENGTH VERSE

" 'I have told you these things, so that in me you may have peace. In this world you will have trouble. But take heart! I have overcome the world.' "
John 16:33

Many of us get half way through life and just burn out. We're worn down and weary by trying to power through on our own might. We lose hope and are broken by the losses we've faced. Jesus clearly tells us in John 16:33 that there will be trials and tribulations in this life, but we need our peace to come from Him alone because He has overcome this fallen world. He also tells us that we can cast all our cares upon Him and have His power to overcome. (1 Peter 5:7 and Psalm 55:22) He will carry us over the finish line with a first place victory. He doesn't want you to settle for the consolation prize just for showing up for the race. I don't know about you, but when I cross that finish line, I want to be at full speed, blazing, with a smile on my face. My deepest desire is to hear, "Job well done, good and faithful servant" from my Lord and Savior, Jesus.

I want you to know this truth. If you started out programmed to fail for whatever reason, or you're just plain out of steam and don't think you can go another step, don't give up. God hasn't given up on you, so don't you give up on yourself. There is still work to be done, and He still has a mighty plan for your life. You have everything you need in Christ to finish stronger than strong!

Soul Strength: the ability through a relationship with God Himself to clearly hear His voice and to receive His wisdom and power that will fill you with joy and direction.

Again we come back to soul strength: the ability through a relationship with God Himself to clearly hear His voice and to receive His wisdom and power that will fill you with joy and direction. Actually, the simple truth is the steps have already been laid out for us. He wrote them down in 66 love letters called the Bible. A large percentage of the population owns a Bible, yet very few look to it for direction. God's Word is the GPS that will lead you directly to soul strength. It contains all the guidance and wisdom needed to live a successful life and finish strong. Allow it access into your mind and your heart, and it will become part of your DNA.

Have you ever tried to carry too much at one time? It wears you down quickly, affects your balance and can be dangerous. Picture a marathon runner with a set of fully packed luggage on his back. It seems ridiculous doesn't it? Yet this is what we do when we try to run the race in our own strength with God-sized loads on our back.

Are you willing to let God lighten your load? Is it your past, a current relationship, a dead-end job? Worry, fear and regret, in particular, are weights far too heavy for us to carry and finish strong. These are not from God and they will disable us. We need to grab hold of hope and trust—they will pull us forward. After a while, all the trophies and titles I won actually became idols to me because I was putting my hope in them to fulfill my heart's desire—something they weren't designed to do. I was missing out on something "great" because I was hanging onto something that was only "good."

STRENGTH BUILDERS

1. What are the idols that are keeping you from finishing strong? Why are they keeping you from finishing strong?

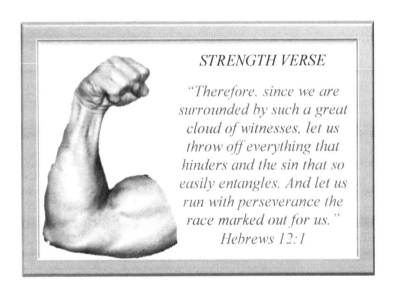

STRENGTH VERSE

"Therefore, since we are surrounded by such a great cloud of witnesses, let us throw off everything that hinders and the sin that so easily entangles. And let us run with perseverance the race marked out for us."
Hebrews 12:1

2. What are some things you hold dear that you haven't surrendered to God?

3. If it were possible to hear the words of your eulogy at your own funeral, what would you like to hear?

4. Make a list of the "good" things that need to be put on hold or eliminated so that "great" can emerge.

5. Imagine crossing God's finish line with a first place victory. Describe the thoughts and feelings that idea evokes.

6. List several ideas that entice you to finish the race strong.

Your Mind: The Ultimate Computer System

A virus that gets into a computer doesn't just happen, it is maliciously put there by someone wanting to do harm. The enemy of your soul wants to plant a virus in your mind. He wants thoughts of past bad decisions, lusts, painful memories of failure and anything negative or harmful to your future to keep playing and playing day and night until they become your identity and the weight that so easily bogs you down.

Let God renew your thought life by prayer and meditating on His Word. He will cast a new vision for your life, one that is pure and filled with the power of truth.

Dreams: Don't Let Them Go, Let Them Grow!

As adults we seem to have a habit of letting go of what is in our heart so we can carry on with what is in our head (all the daily to do items, our job, things that we do almost robotically each day). We seldom stop to ask, "Why am I doing this?" "Is it needed?" "Can I do it differently?" "Is there a better way?" "Am I living out my purpose?" I'm suggesting that it's time to stop and ask.

Children ages 2-7 ask "Why?"

7-17 ask and/or say "Why not?"

Adults say "Just because."

Why is it so fascinating to watch children play? It's because they have no limit on their imagination. They just go for it! Ask a child what he wants to be when he grows up and see what happens. Children don't think small. Astronaut, president, fighter pilot, actress, model, etc.

What happens as we "grow up"? We leave the reality of our dreams and the very unique vision God gave us for our lives behind for "adulthood." Have you ever heard a child say, "I would love to work at a dead end job that I hate and retire broke at

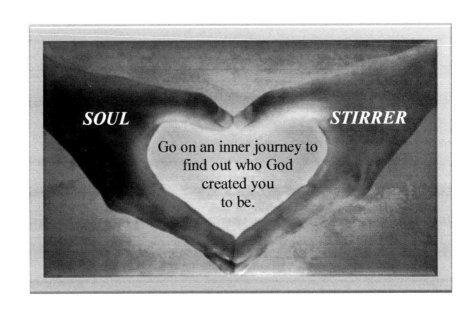

70"? Never! God gives all of us deep heart desires for a reason. Have some fun and go on a mission to dig up those long forgotten dreams. Think like a child for a while! I'm not saying go quit your job tomorrow, but it would be beneficial to take a good look at the dreams that lie deep within you. As you pursue God's direction regarding your dreams, it's possible He may lead you to make some changes in the near future. I know, I know—

we all have responsibilities and families who are relying on us, but imagine them being able to see you at your best. Go on an inner journey to find out who God created you to be. What lights your fire? What brings the most fulfillment? What secret dream haven't you explored yet? What have others said you're great at? I believe you will be pleasantly surprised. Each day is a gift from God, and time is something you cannot get back once it's gone. Go for it and start today!

STRENGTH BUILDERS

1. The toys we played with as a child tell us a lot about the dreams in our heart. What was your favorite toy as a child? Why?

2. What were some of the dreams you had growing up?

3. What passion that once stirred your heart have you let die? Why?

4. Is God asking you to bring it to life and use it for His kingdom? Describe what you're hearing from Him as you pursue Him about the passions He's instilled in you.

Don't Retire, Rewire

Retirement is not biblical. As a matter of fact its way overrated, and may even be deadly. The world's pipe dream is to retire at 60 something, play golf or sit on a boat and do nothing but watch the grandkids run around.

What is the obsession with retirement? Why are we completely worn out just past half-time? Why have we lost hope that there is a better life God wants for us, one that you would never want to retire from? The reality of retirement is that most people live like it's the finish line, but it should be a time when we get our second wind, a time when we can use all the wisdom we've gained from all the hills and valleys of life. The sad truth is most people retire from living.

I smile as I think of a fond memory of Jack saying, "You know, I've never once gotten up in the morning, sat on the end of the bed, and heard God's voice saying, 'Jack, go back and lay down. I'll work out and eat for you.'"

Statistics reveal that when people let their life come to a standstill after retiring, they get a major illness or die within a few years. Retirement was a curse word to my friend and mentor, Jack LaLanne. At 70 years old, Jack was pulling 70 boats across the San Francisco bay. At age 95, he still had a full schedule of seminars, book signings, and was still swimming and doing strength training daily. He was also traveling around the country promoting his Jack LaLanne juicer. Jack died at 96. He ran out of clock long before he ran out of passion and purpose.

No one else can finish this race well for you. I smile as I think of a fond memory of Jack saying, "You know, I've never once gotten up in the morning, sat on the end of the bed, and heard God's voice saying, 'Jack, go back and lay down. I'll work out and eat for you.'" I said this many, many times before, but it's you against you. Get out of your own way, grab onto soul strength and finish the race flourishing in God's unlimited power!

134

STRENGTH BUILDERS

1. What are your current views on retirement?

2. If you are retired, what fills your days?

3. Describe how you think God may lead you to spend your later years in this life?

Identity Theft

The evil one is the original identity thief. He wants your identity to be in titles or accomplishments, things or people. If you have placed your faith in Jesus Christ, your identity is in Him alone. The temporary trophies of this life should not define you. You can never be first place forever, and all that you own, no matter how nice, will someday rust away and be gone forever. The stamp of approval on your life comes from God alone.

Even though you try, you can't compare

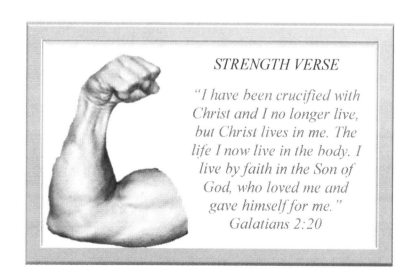

STRENGTH VERSE

"I have been crucified with Christ and I no longer live, but Christ lives in me. The life I now live in the body, I live by faith in the Son of God, who loved me and gave himself for me."
Galatians 2:20

yourself to anybody else because there is no one like you—never has been, never will be. Think about this: there are things on this earth that no one else can accomplish but you. There are seven billion unique individuals on this planet. Most will judge how useful they are and find their worth by looking around to see what everyone else is accomplishing. You need only to look up to get the real answer. If you know Christ, you belong to God and He lives in you.

The life we're living on this earth matters to the God who gave us life! Because God gave us physical bodies, physical fitness is very important! When we take care of our body we are giving thanks to God who gave us our one model year, His amazing temple which is our earthly home.

Financial fitness is also very important! In the New Testament, Jesus spoke more about money than heaven or hell. Why? Because it's a matter of our heart. We are to be good stewards with all the resources He's given us. Everything we do, everything we say, everything we put into our bodies matters to God because it all came from Him and belongs to Him! That's why having soul strength is so vital to finishing strong.

1 Corinthians 10:31, "So whether you eat or drink or whatever you do, do it all for the glory of God."

As we close, I want to remind you of a very important truth in Psalm 90:12: "Teach us to number our days, that we may gain a heart of wisdom." The truth is that none of us knows just how many days we will be given on this earth. The most important thing we can do is invest them in a place and for a cause that is eternal.

I have two final and most important questions for you. They are two that I ask myself and I believe can be an eye opener for how we're doing, how our hearts are, and also about any changes God may want to make in our lives.

STRENGTH BUILDERS

1. If today were your last day, how would God say you finished?

2. What changes will you make to deepen your soul strength and finish strong?

My desire for this workbook is to help you look up to God, dig deep inside your soul, and see yourself through His love and grace. Soul strength is His free gift to you. I want you to be able to give yourself fully to His purpose for your life, and live others-centered, pouring yourself out to a lost and needy world. I never thought the testimony of my trials would change lives all around the world. I am still amazed and humbled that God would take me, an abused and confused, sick child from Brooklyn, along with all of my sin and self-centered ways, and transform my life to be used for His eternal purposes.

God loves to take the tragic and turn it into triumphant. His greatest evidence of this is the cross of Christ. And that is where I'm asking you to turn now. I go back to my life verse, Acts 20:24. The heartbeat of my life is to lead others, whether by testimony, training, seminars or counseling, to a relationship with Jesus, the love of their soul, the living God and the sacrifice for their sins. There is no other way to true joy in your heart or strength for your soul in this life or the next without Jesus as your personal Lord and Savior. Ask Him into your heart today and watch Him transform your very life from the inside out. Look to the one who is hope, who can always be trusted. He is the Father to the fatherless, the one who sacrificed His temple so that you could finish eternally strong. He is the way, the truth, and the life. No one comes to the Father or heaven outside of a relationship with Him and surrender to His Lordship.

I would rather be a slave to Christ in heaven than a free man in this world any day. There are no magic words or formulas to receiving Jesus into your heart. Simply ask Him to be the Lord of your life, and confess that you can't save or change yourself. Salvation is not an emotional decision, or filling out a card and moving on; it's the most important thing you will ever do. Don't continue this walk alone. Please access the links I have provided for help in your journey with Christ.

That will lead to the most complete and fulfilling life

you could ever imagine.

As I said before, you have an enemy who will do everything he can to pull out your roots in Christ before they grow deep. A very powerful but misused verse in God's Word is Psalm 37:4: "Take delight in the Lord, and he will give you the desires of your heart." The only way to have soul strength is that you have to *first* delight in the Lord, and then your heart will be aligned with His to receive and understand His voice. That will lead to the most complete and fulfilling life you could ever imagine. Don't delay in taking delight in Him!

One of the most dangerous words the devil loves to put into our heads is "Tomorrow." Tomorrow I will seek God; tomorrow I will stop doing _____; tomorrow I will finish _____. My friends, *this* is the day to invite Jesus into your heart and make Him the Lord of your life! The truth is, we will all finish someday. How strong we finish and where we go after the earthly race is over comes down to one simple choice God gives us to make. My will be done or Thy will be done? We can choose God or self.

God's voice is speaking to you right now just as He did to me on the Verrazano Bridge. He is speaking to you now just like He did the Israelites when He said, "Today I have given you the choice between life and death, between blessings and curses. Now I call on heaven and earth to witness the choice you make. Oh, that you would choose life, so that you and your descendants might live!" (Deuteronomy 30:19, NLT)

God is asking us to choose life, to choose soul strength, and to choose to finish strong and leave a legacy with His signature on it. As I said in the Introduction to this workbook, Jesus is the true Author of soul strength, and the Author and finisher of my life. My hope is that as you have journeyed with me through this workbook that it has led you toward a beautiful and narrow path that will lead to healing, wholeness and the freedom of soul strength. One way my heart is truly blessed is to hear about the joy of a changed life. I would love for you to send me your personal soul strength story that is either being written or re-written by the Author of life and the Lover of your soul, Jesus.

God bless you.

– Peter

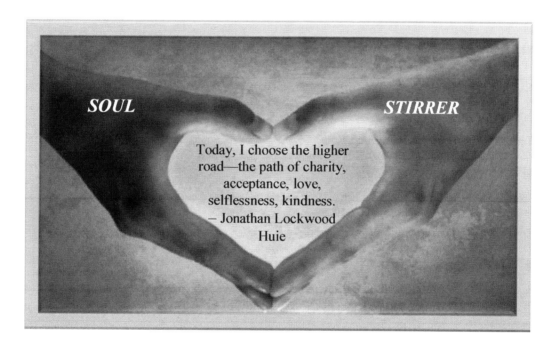

SOUL   STIRRER

Today, I choose the higher road—the path of charity, acceptance, love, selflessness, kindness.
– Jonathan Lockwood Huie

APPENDIX A

History Repeats: *Using two different color wide felt-tip markers, one color for <u>family</u> <u>history</u>, the other color for <u>current events</u>, draw a line from zero out to the degree that the issue occurred or is occurring. If your issue(s) are not in the list, feel free to add your own issues in the blanks provided.*

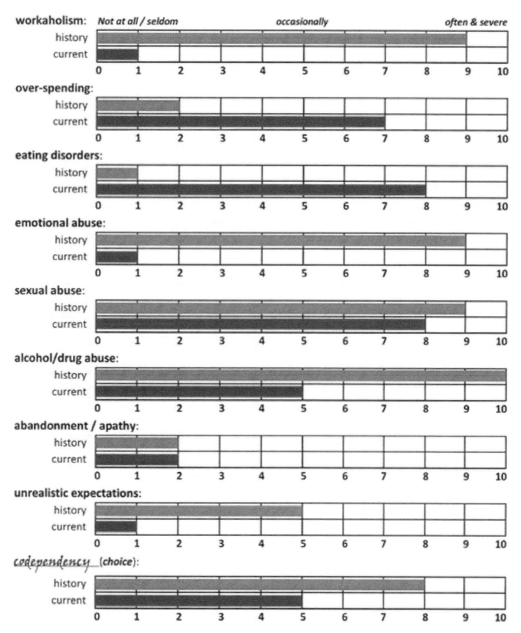

History Repeats: _Using two different color wide felt-tip markers, one color for_ <u>_family_</u> <u>_history_</u>_, the other color for_ <u>_current events_</u>_, draw a line from zero out to the degree that the issue occurred or is occurring. If your issue(s) are not in the list, feel free to add your own issues in the blanks provided._

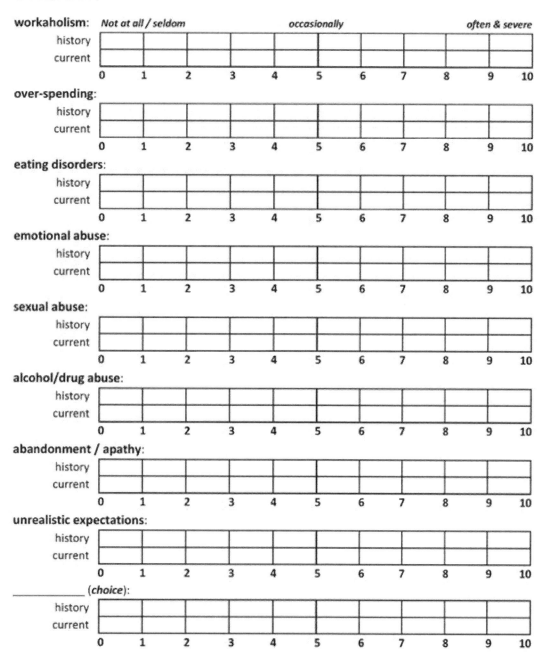

WEEKLY PLANNER

	God / Prayer	Family	Health & Wellness	Rest (Sabbath)	Extended/Spiritual Family & Friends	Work	Hobbies / Fun Time	Other _____
MONDAY	what: from: to:	what: from: to:	what: from: to:	what: from: to:	what: from: to:	what: from: to:	what: from: to:	what: from: to:
TUESDAY	what: from: to:	what: from: to:	what: from: to:	what: from: to:	what: from: to:	what: from: to:	what: from: to:	what: from: to:
WEDNESDAY	what: from: to:	what: from: to:	what: from: to:	what: from: to:	what: from: to:	what: from: to:	what: from: to:	what: from: to:
THURSDAY	what: from: to:	what: from: to:	what: from: to:	what: from: to:	what: from: to:	what: from: to:	what: from: to:	what: from: to:
FRIDAY	what: from: to:	what: from: to:	what: from: to:	what: from: to:	what: from: to:	what: from: to:	what: from: to:	what: from: to:
SATURDAY	what: from: to:	what: from: to:	what: from: to:	what: from: to:	what: from: to:	what: from: to:	what: from: to:	what: from: to:
SUNDAY	what: from: to:	what: from: to:	what: from: to:	what: from: to:	what: from: to:	what: from: to:	what: from: to:	what: from: to:

APPENDIX B

Fueling for Performance

(Excerpt from *Will of Iron* by Peter N. Nielsen)

Nutrition and exercise go hand in hand. What you put in your mouth directly affects what you can do with your body. Most of that picture is the long-range effect. Downing one can of spinach may have helped Popeye lift Bluto off his feet with one arm, but the benefits of good nutrition are not quite that immediate for the rest of us. The "one candy bar equals one winning drive to the basket" that you see in TV commercials is definitely a poor and misrepresented picture of the fuel–performance relationship. Physical performance is all about energy, but it's not about mainlining a blue sports drink to win the NBA playoffs.

Muscles use energy, which they ultimately derive from glucose. The more you use your muscles, the more energy they consume. Sustained exercise of your most important muscle—your heart—will use even more energy. That's why aerobic exercise—putting your heart and lungs into overdrive, fanning the calorie-burning flames with oxygen—will help you trim your body. Assuming, of course, that you're eating right.

Your body can get fuel for exercise from several sources. The most direct source is complex carbohydrates. The digestive system turns carbohydrates into glucose. When this blood sugar is transported to a muscle, it becomes glycogen and is stored there for energy—about 90 minutes' worth. Different kinds of exercise—at different levels of intensity and duration—determine how much energy you use, how quickly you use it, and whether you are burning muscle glycogen, blood glucose, or two secondary sources of energy.

One of these secondary sources (good news) is fat. Depending on the kind of exercise you are performing, exercise *can* burn up fat.

The other source (bad news) is protein. If your body is burning protein for fuel, that means two things: one, you are extremely fatigued, and two, your body is feeding on itself.

Anaerobic exercise is an intense thrust of energy for a matter of 10 to 15 seconds. Traditional weightlifting exercises are anaerobic. Those heavy, quick bursts with the weights build and strengthen muscle, but the anaerobic pathway allows muscles to utilize only one kind of energy: muscle glycogen.

Aerobic exercise elevates the heart rate and sustains it. Generally, it takes 15 or 20 minutes of exercise to get your cardiovascular system up to speed. Spinning, aerobics and kickboxing are just some of the types of classes offered at gyms. And participants are actually burning glucose 18 to 19 times faster than the powerlifter in the next room doing 10 quick presses with a 200-pound barbell. And, as you'll see in a moment, the aerobic exercisers can actually burn up fat—*as long as they don't get too intense in their workout!*

Cross-training, a combination of both aerobic and anaerobic exercise, builds strength *and* endurance. This is a golden pathway to fitness through exercise.

Light to moderate exercise—up to 60 percent of cardiovascular capacity—can be fueled almost entirely through the aerobic pathway. Hormonal changes and decreased insulin output promote the release of fatty acids from fat tissue into the bloodstream. These fatty acids, combined with fat pools in muscle tissue, supply about half the energy for low to moderate exercise. Muscle glycogen and blood glucose supply the rest.

During high intensity exercise—70 percent or more of aerobic capacity—the body does not use fat as fuel. Fat simply can't supply energy fast enough for high intensity exercise, with the body straining to supply enough oxygen to match its workload. Glucose delivers about five calories per liter of oxygen and fat delivers only 4.65 calories, so the body shifts to glucose and glycogen as an energy source. The accumulation of lactic acid is another reason for the shift. Lactic acid, a waste product of high-intensity exercise, hinders mobilization of fatty acids from adipose (fat) tissue.

Duration of exercise also plays a major role in whether or not you burn up any fat in the gym or on the road. Muscle glycogen is the predominant fuel for the first 30 to 60 minutes of most types of exercise. It takes that long for fatty acids to be freed for use as fuel. The longer you exercise, the greater the contribution of fat tissue to your energy consumption. If you exercise moderately for four to six hours, fat can contribute as much as 70 percent of the calories you burn. The longer you exercise, the less intense it must be.

The basic nutritional message is that if burning up fat is one reason you're about to step on a treadmill, you're not interested in blocking or delaying your body's switch to fat as a fuel. *The pre-workout dose of complex carb energy is not the proper strategy for weight loss.*

Ironically, the more fit you are, the easier it is for your body to burn fat. Nobody ever said life was fair. There's scientific proof of this. Endurance training increases an athlete's ability to perform more aerobically during exactly the same exercise—in other words, to use more fat and less glycogen. When I said the body starts to accumulate lactic acid at about 70 percent of its aerobic capacity, I was referring to people well along in a fitness regimen—individuals in training. For an untrained, out-of-shape person, lactic acid starts to accumulate at about 50 percent of aerobic capacity.

This point at which the lactic acid starts building up is called the anaerobic threshold. Increase your anaerobic threshold and you'll increase your ability to burn up fat instead of glycogen. Obviously, your athletic performance in any kind of sustained event will also improve greatly. And there's a double bonus. Trained (fit) individuals also can store about 1½ times as much glycogen in their muscle tissue. So they have more glycogen to begin with and will burn it up at a slower rate.

Even the leanest marathoner stores more body fat than he or she will ever need during exercise. If you're dieting, you have probably figured out by now that your new nutritional lifestyle means you will be burning a lot of glycogen. Right. Your goal is to increase the use of fat as fuel through endurance training, not by eating fat.

CARBOHYDRATES AND PERFORMANCE

Stores of muscle glycogen begin to reach low levels in high intensity exercise that exceeds 90 minutes. When glycogen reaches a critically low supply, the body leaves the athlete two choices: slow the pace dramatically or collapse from exhaustion.

Glycogen can also be depleted in a slow process over several days of repeated heavy training, when you do not eat enough carbohydrates to replace what you've used. When this happens, glycogen stores drop each day—and the athlete wonders why he's not able to maintain his training intensity. That's often the explanation for a "stale" feeling in an exercise program. Instead of the "overtraining" that often gets blamed, it's an insufficiency of carb intake—and sometimes dehydration. That doesn't mean you should eat three baked potatoes at a sitting; it means that your consistent intake of the proper amounts of non-starchy carbs (as well as protein and fat) is critical to performance. Training increases the amount of all nutrition you need, but it is not an excuse to wolf down huge plates of pasta on a daily basis.

(To be specific, if you're in advanced training, we're comparing a 40 percent carbohydrate diet with a 70 percent carbohydrate diet during repeated days of two-hour workouts.)

In one study, fit athletes who started out like gangbusters on an intensive training program were not able to perform even level exercise after seven days on a low-carb diet—with muscle glycogen stores dropping each day.

"Training glycogen depletion," to use the textbook phrase, happens to athletes involved in exercise other than endurance training in the gym. Football, basketball and soccer players—any athlete who uses repeated near-maximum bursts of effort—can experience the same type of exhaustion. Telltale signs are inability to maintain normal exercise intensity and a sudden weight loss of several pounds. Lack of carbohydrate intake and lack of rest days are culprits.

If you are in serious training, you should be eating a diet rich on fibrous complex carbohydrates and you should be taking periodic rest days, during which your muscles will replenish their stores of glycogen. I preach this so much that you'd think the Complex Carb Sales Board was paying me off. But our newest nutritional failing is an onslaught of diet "experts" pushing a "no carb" diet—to counteract our excess intake of empty and starchy carbs. Not only are both approaches dangerous to your health, both leave you unable to exercise properly.

And one more word about simple vs. complex carbs. Yes, simple carbs also provide glycogen synthesis. But fibrous, unprocessed, complex carbs provide more nutrition—including fiber, iron and B complex vitamins necessary for metabolism. Most importantly, the "good" complex carbs are time-released and will not turn to fat if not burned up immediately. My own recommendation is a non-training diet of 45 to 55 percent carbohydrates—of which 10 percent can be simple carbs from fruits and juices and 10 percent from starches.

CARB INTAKE BEFORE EXERCISING

While you are exercising or performing athletically, the body relies on pre-existing glycogen or fat storage for energy. A pre-exercise meal or snack won't do anything for you immediately, but the carbohydrates can add to blood glucose—and energy—if you exercise for more than an hour. That's why athletes who compete in a prolonged endurance event that relies heavily on blood sugar won't perform as well if they skip breakfast. The overnight fast lowers their liver glycogen storage, the main source of blood sugar.

In the past, athletes have been discouraged from eating on the morning before training or a competition. Common advice is to eat two to three hours before exercising, so if there's a morning track meet or an early appointment at the gym, most people will skip breakfast. The rationale is that any food remaining in the stomach at the start of exercise might nauseate you when blood is diverted from the gastrointestinal tract to the exercising muscle. Athletes also have been advised to avoid high-carbohydrate meals immediately before training on the grounds that higher insulin levels might cause hypoglycemia or fatigue. Actually, there is a great range of personal reaction here. Some athletes in endurance training are insensitive to lowered blood sugars (I'm one of them). There's really no substitute for experimenting with your own body's reaction to pre-exercise meals.

The simple fact is that eating before exercise can help restore depleted liver and muscle glycogen storage. If gastric emptying is a concern, then you can always try a commercial liquid meal. They're high in carbohydrate calories, contribute to hydration and can be consumed nearer to the time of a competition because of the shorter gastric emptying time. They may help *prevent* pre-event nausea in a tense athlete. Liquid meals also are more convenient during daylong competitions, such as track meets, triathlons or tennis tournaments. Just remember to include your proper balance of protein and fat as well.

How much carbohydrate should an athlete eat before an event? The consensus suggests one to four grams per kilogram of bodyweight, consumed one to four hours before exercising. To prevent possible gastro distress, decrease the intake if you eat nearer to the time of the event—four grams per kilo of bodyweight four hours prior to the event, down to one gram one hour prior to the event.

Good examples of pre-exercise carbohydrate foods: oatmeal, fruits, juices and non-fat yogurt.

What about consuming simple sugar before exercise? Studies on the subject are all over the map. For sure, consuming a candy bar before anaerobic exercise—such as weight training—will not increase performance because your body already has plenty of glycogen stored for the activity. It could be useful, however, for a long-distance runner who will need energy when muscle glycogen falls to a low level. Again, there are great individual differences here. You should test your own reaction in training.

FLUID INTAKE BEFORE EXERCISE

For peak performance, you should be fully hydrated before training or competing. Drink 16 to 20 ounces of water through the two hours before training, and drink another 16 ounces of cold fluid 10 to 15 minutes before starting.

Drinking the full quota of fluids just before exercise can produce hyperhydration. Some people think hyperhydrating improves thermoregulation by shortening the usual delay in sweating and decreasing the quantity of sweat. No serious advantages have been proven for this strategy, however. Particularly in hot weather, I'd suggest an athlete should drink no more fluid—probably about 20 ounces—than he or she will be comfortable with.

What kind of fluid? More than 15 minutes before exercising, stick with water. In the final 15 minutes, water-diluted fruit juice or a sports drink is a good choice if the activity will be longer than an hour.

I shouldn't have to tell you that caffeine is a lousy pre-exercise beverage.

FLUID INTAKE DURING EXERCISE

Individual responses vary tremendously. Drinking fluids during exercise is as much an art as a science, even though there are tons of reports on the subject. In any case, fluid replacement during exercise—training or competition—is vital to prevent thermal damage. In training it helps you get into a routine for drinking fluids during competition.

You should aim to replace at least 50 percent of fluid loss while you exercise. Drink four to six ounces of fluid every 10 to 15 minutes. Cold fluid (40 to 50 degrees Fahrenheit) will help cool the core body temperature and will leave the stomach more rapidly than warm fluid. Warmer fluids make sense if you're exercising in cool or cold weather.

The idea is to replace lost fluids, so one of the prime attributes in choosing a drink is that you find it palatable. If you like it, you'll drink it. Water is palatable to most anyone. Water also is inexpensive and easily absorbed. Good stuff, that water.

Sports drinks combine glucose and sodium to promote rapid absorption from the small intestine. That's OK. Just remember that any benefits of carb replacement are strictly limited to endurance activities. If you drink juice, it should be diluted at least by half.

CARBOHYDRATES AFTER EXERCISE

You know that eating adequate amounts of carbohydrate during intensive training is vital to replenish muscle glycogen stores. The time period when you eat after exercise is also important. The sooner the better.

The only serious study I've found on the subject measured muscle glycogen production when two grams of carbohydrates per kilogram of body weight were consumed immediately after exercise, two hours after exercise and four hours after exercise. Two hours after exercise, glycogen production was cut by a third. Four hours after exercise it was cut by 45 percent.

There are several possible explanations. Blood flow to the muscle is greater immediately after exercise. Muscle cell is more receptive to glycogen. And the cells are more sensitive to insulin, which promotes glycogen production.

Commercial complex carb drinks can make sense here, because many athletes are not hungry for a meal after heavy exercise.

How much should you consume after heavy exercise? The best evidence suggests about 400 calories (or 100 grams) of carbs within 15 minutes of a workout, but you still have to get your protein and a little fat somewhere.

FLUID INTAKE AFTER EXERCISE

Intensive exercise blunts the sensation of thirst, and it will be quenched before you replace the fluids you have lost in a workout or competition. That's why you've got to be deliberate about fluid replacement after your event or workout. For every pound of bodyweight lost, you should drink about 16 ounces of liquid. Start drinking as soon as the workout is over—even before you shower—then keep drinking at a comfortable pace.

The temperature of what you drink is less important at this point, but a warm drink can prevent hypothermia on a cold day of outdoor activity.

If you undertake moderate exercise in moderate temperature, you're going to lose more water than electrolytes—meaning water is the crucial nutrient to replace. Plain water is fine. A sweet-tasting fluid has only the side benefit of stimulating you to drink more. Alcohol or caffeine—in coffee or soda pop—are diuretics, and will only make you lose more water.

Fluid replacement generally follows the same principles no matter what your activity, but some sports need special consideration. Fluid should never be restricted for football players, for example. In hot weather, exercising underneath all that gear can generate incredible fluid loss. Endurance runners and cyclists must drink fluid while running or pedaling. Protecting against dehydration is such an important factor that runners and cyclists must learn to function with fluid in their stomachs, even if it's a personal discomfort. Swimmers—who bury themselves in water—lose pounds of the stuff while sitting around in the sunshine between events.

In some quarters, two particular sports raise fluid deprivation to a near-criminal level. Boxing and wrestling are based on weight classifications, and the easiest way to make weight is to shed water. It's dangerous and stupid.

Water plays a key role in athletic performance by maintaining blood volume, which is necessary for cardiovascular function and for regulating body temperature. Thirst is an unreliable barometer of your hydration. That's why athletes—and recreational competitors—should follow the guidelines above.

Fluid replacement is even more important with the very young and the very old.

Children have lower heat tolerance, a lower sweating capacity and a lower cardiac output—which makes it harder to dissipate excess body heat. In cold temperatures, their extremities are more likely to freeze. Kids should drink 10 to 14 ounces of fluid before going out to play. I know it sounds impractical, but a boy or girl playing in warm temperatures should continue to replace fluids at the rate of about three ounces every 10 to 15 minutes during activity.

As for older people, one survey found that after 24 hours of fluid deprivation, 67- to 75-year-old men were less thirsty and drank less water than 20- to 31-year-old men. Besides which, many older people are taking many medications—often including diuretics. Fluid consumption needs to be carefully monitored as we grow older.

The Building Block to Muscle

(Excerpt from *Will of Iron* by Peter N. Nielsen)

Protein is the royalty of nutrients. It is found in some of our highest-priced foods. (It's also found in some of our lowest-priced foods, but they tend to get snubbed—as if you couldn't possibly find a *protein* living at that address.) Many people eat unhealthy meals every day, confident they are doing themselves a favor because they are loading up on protein. It is, after all, the stuff that builds muscle.

Several generations were raised on nutritional folklore that went something like: "Protein is real food; the rest of it is junk and fattening."

The fact is, protein *is* the royalty of nutrients. But to have a healthy relationship with protein you must treat it like royalty. Protein has a very limited schedule, and you must accommodate it. If you are building muscle, through weightlifting or otherwise, you absolutely must take a scientific approach to protein consumption. Otherwise, you will be tearing yourself apart when you think you are building yourself up.

Anaerobic exercise *breaks down* muscle tissue. Your musculature then replaces itself with larger, stronger tissue—if you are consuming the proper amount of protein *at the right time.* Since the body can utilize just 35 to 40 grams of protein in any 2½ hour period, sitting down and gorging yourself on protein will produce nothing but fat and toxic wastes. So the amount of protein you consume through the day must be carefully adjusted to fit your exercise regimen. The more muscle you tear down, the more protein you need to replace it. The less you exercise, the more you need a commonsense diet of complex carbohydrates.

This protein connection also often explains why crash diets fail—or even boomerang—leaving the puzzled dieter weighing more than he or she did in the first place.

A tremendous lowering of caloric intake for an extended period lowers the basal metabolism rate (BMR), making it difficult if not impossible to continue shedding body fat. If you foolishly go on a starvation diet while exercising, and deprive yourself of protein, you will lose muscle instead of fat. I can guarantee you that losing muscle will not produce a great loss in size—just a lowering of your metabolism and tone.

While in training, it is absolutely essential that you can eat *four, five or even six meals* a day—not just for the other nutritional benefits of that regimen that we have talked about, but to get protein to your muscles. If you eat more than 40 grams of protein in any 2½ hour period, you might as well be pouring the precious stuff out on your driveway.

So what's an accurate, practical way of selecting and monitoring your protein intake? How much protein is enough?

You'll read advice ranging from one-half gram of protein to a full gram of protein per pound of body weight—a 100 percent variance!

The chart at the end of this chapter—multiplying your ideal body weight by your activity load—tells what's right for you.

I use exactly the same formula. Because I'm a bodybuilder in training and do a tremendous amount of intense anaerobic exercise, I need a large amount of protein. The way I get it is by eating six carefully planned meals a day, none of which look like anything out of a Norman Rockwell Thanksgiving scene. This is the *only* way I can get the protein I need. It *must* be spaced through the day.

If you're a weightlifter, or training intensively in another sport, you can follow my program out the window and benefit greatly. If you exercise moderately, lightly, or not at all, this will strike you as one bizarre-looking regimen. But remember, my goal here is not to get every reader eating chicken breasts three or four times a day. It's for you to understand how the body accepts protein, and how you must incorporate that into your own nutrition regimen—whatever your physical workload.

How to Determine

Daily Protein Requirement

GRAMS OF PROTEIN PER DAY, DEPENDING ON ACTIVITY LEVEL

(Multiply by ideal body weight, using chart below.)

.5 grams per lb.:   Sedentary, no sports or fitness training

.6 grams per lb.:   Jogger or in light fitness training

.7 grams per lb.:   Sports participant or moderate training three days a week

.8 grams per lb.:   Moderate training every day, aerobic or weights

.9 grams per lb.:   Heavy weight training daily

1.0 grams per lb.: Heavy weight training daily plus sports training, or two-a-day
    weight training

Ideal Body Weight	Total Daily Protein Grams					
	.5	.6	.7	.8	.9	1.0
90	45	54	63	72	81	90
100	50	60	70	80	90	100
110	55	66	77	88	99	110
120	60	72	84	96	108	120
130	65	78	91	104	117	130
140	70	84	98	112	126	140
150	75	90	105	120	135	150
160	80	96	112	128	144	160
170	85	102	119	136	153	170
180	90	108	126	144	162	180
190	95	114	133	152	171	190
200	100	120	140	160	180	200
210	105	126	147	168	189	210
220	110	132	154	176	198	220
230	115	130	161	184	207	230
240	120	144	168	192	216	240

As a pro bodybuilder, here's how I use the same protein guidelines that you can adapt from the chart:

Let's say 190 is my ideal body weight. If I were not involved in sports whatsoever—didn't even jog—I would need protein by a factor of .5 grams times 190, or 95 grams of protein a day. If I were into jogging—or light fitness, training maybe once a week—I would need .6 grams of protein times 190 (114 grams of protein a day). Training three times a week, I would need .7 grams (133 grams total). Training daily with weights or aerobics on a moderate basis, I would need .8 grams (152 grams total). And if I were into heavy weight training every day, I would need .9 grams (171 total). In the last 12 weeks before a competition, doing a double split of exercises, I would need one full gram per pound of ideal body weight—or 190 grams of protein a day.

At 27 grams per average boneless, skinless chicken breast, and three grams per one large egg white, and 30 grams per typical broiled unbreaded fish filet, we're talking about a lot of chow. You might literally get tired of eating. In that case, to reach your quotas, you'll probably want to supplement your food with egg white powder or commercial amino acid powders. (As always, you shouldn't drink water from 15 minutes before a meal until 30 to 60 minutes afterward, or you'll have absorption problems.)

I carry a log with me and keep close track of those protein grams, and the time that I consume them.

If your protein intake matches your needs and your fat intake is low, you are doing exactly what is needed on the nutritional side to acquire tremendous muscle definition. The muscles you break down anaerobically come back bigger and stronger with the aid of your careful protein intake.

In the fall of 1991, I saw a tremendous difference in my own body from the Southeastern USA competition to the Mr. World competition. My body fat was 4 or 5 percent for the USA on October 5, and on November 23 it was 2.5 percent for the Mr. World. What I did was increase my protein intake from .75 gram to one full gram per pound of ideal body weight. At the Mr. World I had more size, more "cut" and had less fat on my body.

Don't forget: This didn't happen because I guzzled protein. It happened because my protein intake matched my very heavy training load, and was spaced so that my body could use it.

You Gotta Have Heart

The Basics about Cardiovascular Conditioning

(Excerpt from *Will of Iron* by Peter N. Nielsen)

Let's take a look at the average out-of-shape driver whose air-conditioned cocoon blows a tire on the freeway. The suit coat comes off, the sleeves get rolled up, the jack comes out of the trunk. In a few minutes, our friend is going to get a double whammy. He is going to discover that he is seriously lacking in both kinds of fitness—endurance and strength.

Soon after lugging the spare out of the trunk and squatting down to yank on the lug wrench, he's sucking wind. Aerobically speaking, his cardiovascular endurance is about equal to the Happy 40th Birthday balloon that has been hanging around—barely—for a couple of weeks.

Then, trying to twist the fifth lug nut, he finds that right at the moment he probably couldn't twist the top off a pop bottle. His *strength*—something built up anaerobically through resistance against muscle, whether by weights pumped in the gym or by boxes unloaded from a truck—is non-existent.

There, in a graphic nutshell, you see some obvious reasons for conditioning your body along both fitness paths. Aerobics training and resistance training are two entirely different animals, but in the real world they go together like country and western. (Remember, we don't talk ham and eggs on our new dietary regimen.) Aerobics and anaerobics. Endurance and strength. Work on them both in a conditioning program and you can say that you're into "cross-training."

Imagine, for example, that you have worked yourself up to a three-day-a-week regimen—in your own basement—of 20 minutes of jump rope or hula hoop (aerobics), followed by a Dynaband routine (anaerobics). That would make you as solidly into cross-training as if you had a personal trainer and access to a million-dollar gym.

For starters, you need to know something about aerobics. If you really are at a starting point, losing fat is undoubtedly one of your goals. Aerobic exercise is the fat-burning king. You could go dancing with your spouse and –assuming you stayed on your feet and the tempo stayed up—you could boogie off 600 calories in a very aerobic evening. An hour of working your way through a weight-lifting routine—even if you powerlifted the Empire State Building—would burn off practically zilch.

The fat-burning qualities of aerobics is an attention-getter for couch potatoes. But the real reason for pursuing aerobic fitness is what it does for the heart. Aerobics, in fact, strengthens the entire cardiovascular system. More oxygen gets to the cells that need it, and it becomes easier for your heart to get it there. An aerobically fit individual's heart beats about 17 million fewer times in the course of a year. You don't need to be a physiologist to understand what that means.

In terms of performance, the big fringe benefit is endurance. We've got quite an endurance range in this crazy modern world where exercise is something we have to schedule into our lives. The air-sucking tire changer, for example, might be a salesman who works right across the desk from a marathoner. Both of them good people, both of them kind to their spouses and children, both of them wearing $1,000 suits, both of them driving big new cars. But one of them can run 26 miles and one of them can't change a tire. The wild thing is that I'm not exaggerating the comparison for effect. You'll find that exact Mutt and Jeff duo in the real world, in almost any office.

So what does Mutt have to do to get into some kind of cardiovascular reality zone, besides taking remote controls out of his life? Specifically, he should exercise aerobically three or four days a week, keeping his heart at its ideal target rate for at least 20 to 30 minutes. Here's what that's about.

Put two fingers on your wrist and take a pulse for 10 seconds. Multiply by six. That's your *resting heart rate*.

If you're a woman or an out-of-shape man, subtract your age from 220.

If you're a man in very fit condition, subtract half your age from 205. That's a calculation of your *maximum heart rate*.

168

An aerobic exercise program means that you take your heart to its ideal target rate, sustain it there for a certain period of time, and do the workout a certain number of times per week. Different authorities suggest slightly different numbers for all those variables. The ones I follow are the American Heart Association (the ideal target rate of 60 to 70 percent of maximum) and the Institute for Aerobic Research (four times a week, 20 minutes per session; or three times a week, 30 minutes a session).

What's going on while you exercise aerobically? Your blood becomes more oxygen-rich, and at the same time removes more carbon dioxide from all your body's cells after delivering the oxygen. Your muscle cells become more efficient at processing oxygen and eliminating lactic acid (meaning you won't have the lactic acid soreness that follows anaerobic exercise). Your blood vessels become more flexible, so your heart is less taxed. Lung capacity increases. Your heart, itself a muscle, becomes better supplied with blood and grows stronger. Your supply of HDL (good) cholesterol increases. While the supply of LDL (bad cholesterol) decreases.

And then there's your resting heart rate. An unconditioned person's heart may beat as much as 80 times a minute *at rest*. A person with good cardiovascular fitness will have a resting heart rate of 45 to 50 beats a minute. A superbly conditioned endurance athlete might have a resting rate in the range of 40 beats per minute.

Meanwhile, as we said when discussing nutrition, your basal metabolism rate stays higher even *after* aerobic exercise. So there you sit, burning calories and asking less of your heart. The beer commercials have it all wrong. It doesn't get any better than this.

If you work out too hard, you cross that anaerobic threshold. The heart loses all that efficiency in delivering oxygen and carting away carbon dioxide. You are no longer endurance training, and you will—in fact—have no endurance. You'll slow down, or quit, from exhaustion.

As your cardiovascular system becomes more fit, your anaerobic threshold will rise. More fit individuals can train at 75 to 80 percent of their maximum heart rate. Exceptionally fit individuals might even be able to train aerobically above 80 percent. Physiologists can determine your threshold with a treadmill test. The two-finger pulse check and the 60 to 70 percent target rate will work fine for starters. It's important to keep tab of your pulse, though, because you don't want to work yourself beyond the anaerobic threshold. It's not a health-threatening line if you cross it; but it will mean a quick end to the aerobic effect, and a quick end to your workout. (By the way, we'll remind you that you should get a physical exam before launching any fitness regimen after a long period of inactivity.)

You can do specific aerobic exercises in the gym, or in your living room. But *any* exercise that takes your heart to its ideal target rate. Sustains it and doesn't cross the anaerobic threshold is aerobic exercise. A long, brisk walk in your Levi's, bringing your dog along for *his* exercise, is just as aerobic as running in place in designer tights while watching a $50 exercise [video]. Jogging is one of the all-time great aerobic exercise. Many sports and activities, as we'll see in a minute, spill over—in varying degrees—to that gray area of cross-training.

Anaerobic exercise (literally "without oxygen") involves a quick, maximum thrust of energy. Aerobic exercise is a sustained, plodding activity in which the heart is stoking up the body with oxygen and burning up energy. Anaerobic exercise is a burst of effort that cannot possibly be sustained. Sprinting is anaerobic. Jogging is aerobic. Doing 10 bench presses with a heavy barbell is anaerobic. Dancing like a kid through your living room is aerobic. When you provide *resistance* against the sustained burst of effort, you are building muscle. Resistance is relative. Two hundred pounds of iron disks, for example, is stone cold resistance. The sets of exercises that make up a weightlifting routine are pure anaerobic resistance training. Don't tell a sprinter, however, that he is encountering no resistance when he drives off the starting blocks and pushes his body forward for 50 incredibly tense meters, trying to improve his time by a few hundredths of a second. His thighs will tell him there is resistance. (You could set a world dash record, by the way, without getting in a lick of aerobic exercise; at least not in the running of the race.)

A swimmer doing laps in relatively leisurely fashion is getting a first-class aerobic workout. A swimmer dashing a lap is not exercising aerobically. He is, however, encountering real resistance from the water with every stroke. Put a pair of those floppy leather mitts on his hands and he'd be meeting resistance equal to a modest dumbbell.

Cross-country skiing is excellent aerobic exercise. Ask anybody who has tried it about the uphills, though. Plenty of resistance there.

So there is haphazard cross-training in most any recreational sport that involves sustained physical exertion and bursts of maximum effort. It is, however, just that: haphazard. And generally not very symmetrical. The thighs of speed skater would be one good example. You generally can get aerobically fit by "going out to play." Anaerobic conditioning is more tricky. A full-body resistance training program is the only way to systematically strengthen muscles in all the body parts. For that matter, specific resistance exercises are the best way to strengthen any particular muscles that need extra work. That's why athletes from football, basketball, hockey—dozens of entirely different sports—head to the gym for conditioning.

An inactive person most definitely wants to get his or her conditioning program started with aerobics. Burn that fat. Strengthen that heart. Get that BMR raised. The benefits are all pretty obvious. Aerobics is the *core* of turning a flabby society into a fit society. It *will* tone muscle. Strength can be built in various individual and team sports. If the whole country were riding bicycles and rowing and playing soccer, I'd be deliriously happy. But it should be no great surprise to learn that I believe almost anyone can benefit from weight training, if they choose to try it. Most people would rather cut the grass or clean out the cat's litter box. I think an amazing number would change their minds if they got into lifting.

What are the benefits?

First of all, if you're looking to build muscle, the weight room is the best place to be. No other game or sport that I know of directs work exactly to the muscles that need it, parcels out the work within a brief period of time and puts you entirely in command of what happens to your body. We've come a long way just within my lifetime in terms of working a weight program into a total fitness concept. Instead of going into the gym and jerking macho poundage a few reps at a time, we warm up and cool down aerobically. The power-lifting branch of the sport still measures life by how many pounds they can put in the air, but most of us think in terms of overall strength, endurance and muscle tone.

Which leads us to the cosmetic fringe benefit. That applies to aerobics as well, of course, because cosmetic step one is to shed the fat. Cosmetic step two—the one that crosses the T's and dots the I's—is to replace the fat with some solid lean tissue. I keep saying this is the least important reason to be fit. But we do live in a Vogue and GQ world.

The pressures to look our best are intense. Besides, firming up the body does wonders for mental health. It's a whole lot healthier and cheaper than plastic surgery. And it will give an excuse—a necessity—for buying some new clothes.

Back on a more important vein, don't let that buzzword "strength" get in the way of your thinking. "Strength" doesn't mean you're a musclehead. It takes strength to carry a briefcase and a sample kit to a dozen appointments a day. It takes strength to clean house. Our friend discovered it takes strength to change a tire. It takes strength *to get up out of a chair*. Strength is part of everyday life. Your cardiovascular system and your muscles deteriorate every day you're inactive. Every *year* that you're inactive, the toll gets more serious. Until finally, a minor little unfamiliar movement pops a muscle or tendon somewhere. Aches and pains often are a body's way of saying: "I've got no strength." Weight training is a good way to answer: "Here you are."

If you already are an active person, if you are an athlete, that's all the more reason to become a lifter. I've trained pro athletes from every type of sport. All of them need specific strengths, and there's a way of improving performance in any sport through a specific weight program. A football linebacker basically needs to be able to push cattle around. A basketball player needs to protect and improve his already incredible leaping ability. Hockey players fly down the ice, but they need tremendous upper body strength to win those shoving matches in the corners. I trained a college quarterback known for his agility and flexibility. He was obviously not interested in bulking up with a heavy-duty anaerobic program. But he needed to keep his legs strong, and a program of supersets increased his endurance.

In other words, weight training—for all this talk about muscle—is meant to help you get to the point where you don't even have to *think* about your muscles. It's a way of getting ready for life's combat, whatever that might be: knocking down a lineman, changing a tire, cleaning a house, rehabilitating an injury. Weights—and other forms of resistance training—are a piece of overall fitness and well-being. Some bodybuilders become obsessed with it, for sure. But have you talked to any golfers lately? You tell me which is the healthier obsession: tapping a little white ball or building muscle?

The fact is, most fit people that I know in daily life away from the gym play racquetball or swim or play tennis. They walk a lot. What resistance training they do is with Dynabands and 10-pound dumbbells. They are at an advanced state of aerobic fitness, and that's where they want to be.

That's fine. Weights aren't for everyone.

But as you design a new lifetime nutrition and exercise path, kick a few tires. You don't buy a new car without checking out all the models and options, and your body is a lot more important than a new car. A health club isn't a bad place to start, even if you ultimately take your act back out on the road. A good club offers both aerobic and anaerobic options and has qualified staff to help you choose a path that works for you. A bad club will burn your money and waste your time.

If you can afford it, if you find the idea of going to a club to be a motivating factor for fitness, and if you want to test the various waters, here's a checklist of factors for choosing a club. Some of them may seem obvious, but I've seen every one of them turn out to be the difference between a good and bad choice.

• Is the club open when workouts will fit your schedule? If so, find out whether it has kept those hours long enough to suggest they won't change next month.

• Is it near your home or office? Ten miles might not seem like much in your initial enthusiasm. But what about two months from now when you're dragging after a hard day and it's time for your workout?

• What can you afford? Cost of membership varies widely. Some clubs have family plans at reduced rates. Many offer occasional specials for new members. If this is strictly a test drive, availability of a short-term membership might be a big factor.

• What about general upkeep? Are weight machines in good working order? Are the locker rooms clean? Take a good look around the place. If you don't want to be there today, you certainly won't want to be there in six weeks.

• How well-equipped is the club? Are there plenty of aerobics devices, such as treadmills, bikes, and studios for aerobics, spinning, or kickboxing? Is the floor of the aerobics studio shock-compensated? Is there an adequate number of strength developing devices, including weight machines and free weights? Anywhere you have to wait for time with a device is a bad place to work out. You don't want to live there. You want to get in, have an intense training session, and get out.

• Is there at least one exercise physiologist on staff who is certified by American College of Sports Medicine? It's important to have someone on hand who knows how to instruct you instead of just looking pretty.

• Are staff members certified in CPR? That's not meant to scare you. It's just another little sign that management is on its toes.

• Does it offer programs that interest you? Some clubs, for example, emphasize racquet sports. If you don't play racquet sports, you won't much care. The same applies to a swimming pool, which can account for a big piece of your membership fee.

• Are you looking for a place to meet friends, as well as to exercise? If so, does it offer a place for socializing?

• How much individual attention will you get? Is personal training offered? Will an exercise program be customized for your needs? Will it cost extra?

• Which items—massage, manicure, personal training, tanning, dining facilities, juice bar, etc.—are *a la carte* and which come with the club?

• Do you know someone who is already a member? If so, ask him or her to rate the club. If you're lucky enough to have this option, it's one of the best barometers.

• Beware of the gyms staffed by overly sculptured employees who are too busy staring at their own reflections in the mirror to help you find your way around. That isn't a physique; that's a musclehead.

• Visit several clubs and ask for a tour. Make all of your visits on a day and at a time when you would be likely to be working out. It'll give you a true sense of traffic. The same club that looks uncrowded at 10 a.m. might be a zoo at 5:30 p.m.—after work, and just when you'd normally be showing up.

• Don't join any club without first trying out the facilities. Many will let you do so free of charge, at least for one visit. If not, it's worth paying the one-time rate.

Some people have the discipline and enough knowledge or self-study prowess to get a genuine conditioning program up and running at home, on their own. Some people don't. If you fall in the latter group, don't be one of the thousands of people who don't try a club because they're embarrassed by their flabby bodies. This is where shopping around and kicking tires becomes vitally important. Clubs have diverse clientele just like bars and restaurants. You don't, obviously, want to be in a power-lifters' gym. But you also don't want to be in a pleasant, attractive room where the emphasis is on socializing rather than fitness. Look and you'll find a place that meets a happy medium.

And, trust me, half the people in the place were wary, if not terrified, the first time they showed up for a workout. That feeling will disappear, along with the flab and the aches and pains.

Anatomy of a Workout

(Excerpt from *Will of Iron* by Peter N. Nielsen)

They don't call it a "routine" for nothing. An exercise program requires discipline of structure. Patterns in choosing the exercises themselves. Safety precautions. Warmup and cooldown. When you're doing the actual work, you're doing *repetitions*, or reps.

It all sounds so dreary. To be honest, on some days, it *can* be dreary. Being fit doesn't mean you're emotionless, or that your biorhythms somehow hum into a single, glowing groove. One day you'll go into the gym or into the basement full of physical and mental energy. Another day, you'll be drained. It could be for a thousand reasons. You had an argument with your spouse or significant other; it was your birthday yesterday, and you made a serious departure from your nutrition regimen; you have a cold; your boss told you this morning that your paperwork was moving too slow; you're in the 10th week of a hurry-up, tight-deadline, 10-week project. Every day in your life is not the same.

Certain aspects of your fitness program, however, *are* the same, every time. Don't look at it as dreariness. Look at it as something dependable in an undependable world. Or as order amid chaos. Look at it as what a great musician, who performs to cheering crowds in concert halls around the world, does behind the scenes. Except that you've got it made compared to the great musician. Everything is turned around backwards in your favor. For every minute he's on stage, he has practiced scales for hours on end. For every week you're on stage, you spend just a few hours in the gym. You're practicing for *life*.

We're going to talk in this chapter about some of the basic elements and principles that make up a solid, safe, productive workout. We'll talk in terms of being in the gym, but you'll see that 90 percent of these pointers will apply if you're working out in your basement. We'll talk in terms of weight training, but you'll also see that 90 percent of what I say also applies to Dynabands and calisthenics and broomsticks and towels. These are the nuts and bolts of working out, and they are the same whether you are taking your first baby steps to fitness, or you've been pumping iron since gyms were invented.

PARTNERS

You can get fit, or sculpt your body to the best it can be, without ever once using a workout partner. But, man, is it easier—and safer—if you do the job two-by-two. I strongly recommend that everyone find a partner for his or her workout. A regular partner, of course, is the best.

Why is it best? For common-sense reasons.

Competition breeds success. This does *not* mean that when you enter the gym it's the bottom of the ninth, two outs, bases loaded and you're the batter. It's not a *pressure* thing, it's a *motivational* thing. When that last set, or those ninth and 10th reps, require a little extra digging, it helps to have someone—even a friendly someone—on hand to see whether or not you do the work. (You're there for him or her, too, of course.) Don't forget that your partner is also in a "me vs. me" competition. He knows that it's not a question of whether you press 500 pounds, but how you stack up against yourself. When you make it through a routine with a 110-pound bar for the first time, you can *show off!* It works at every level—beginner or advanced. It's, "Look, Ma. No hands!" It's just plain psychological common sense.

Then there is what you might call the honesty factor. Not that I could accuse you of cheating. I certainly would never accuse anyone of cheating at golf, which is by reputation the most honorable of games. But how many strokes, on average, do you suppose we should add to all scorecards of golfers who play a round on their own?

Partners are a first-class safety factor. It's very much like swimming alone versus having a "buddy." You get cramps, or hit a sudden wall of fatigue, and somebody's there to bail you out. In weight training, it's called "getting stuck." People have been seriously injured, or killed, when they got stuck with hundreds of pounds of iron raised above their neck. I really don't recommend anyone *ever* working with heavy weights unless they have a partner. And common sense suggests that anyone undertaking heavy exertion of any kind should at least have someone else in sight in case they become distressed in any way. (Safety should be a concern in *any* kind of exercise. Cyclists, for example, should wear a helmet. If you don't, try this one on for size: *Football players* are smart enough to wear helmets.)

Finally, it's more fun to work out with a partner. It's like the difference between shooting hoops by yourself, or having a little game of one-on-one.

WARMUPS AND COOLDOWNS

A smart person doesn't hop into a $50,000 car on a cold February morning, start the engine and immediately see how quickly they can get from zero to 80 m.p.h. You don't do that to your body, either.

Warmups and cooldowns are a vital part of a routine, whether you are doing towel pulls in your dining room or pumping 300 pounds on a lat machine at the gym. Even if your entire routine consists of two songs' worth of hula hoop, you should begin and end with a few minutes of running in place, holding your arms out from your sides and wriggling them to loosen them up.

Get your heart rate up and get more blood in the muscles. Get your breathing up to speed. In the gym before a workout, do three to five minutes of a nice, even, slow-to-medium pace on an aerobics device—a stationary bike, a treadmill, or a stair machine.

Then do a few minutes of stretches. Muscles and tendons and ligaments can do an incredible amount of work. But do them a favor and help their elasticity—ease into it. It'll help prevent snapping and tearing when you get to the heavier part of your routine. There are a zillion stretches and many philosophies of stretching. A lot of it is idiosyncratic—meaning you find what's best for you. Make it a part of your self-education—from books and magazines, from personnel at your gym, from training partners, from self-experiment.

At the end of your workout, reverse the process. Do a couple minutes of stretches, then do 3 to 5 minutes of aerobic cooldown.

During your resistance-training workout itself, do a specific warmup for each exercise. In essence, do a super-light set (it doesn't count in your log or diary) that previews the movements for the muscle you are going to exercise. If it's a set of bench presses, for example, do a warmup set with just the bar, and no weights.

BREATHING

Key organs of the human body have all kinds of backup capacity that most people don't use. Being your best sometimes means tapping into this reserve. We use only a minuscule part of our brainpower, for instance. And the average person uses only about a quarter of his lung capacity. When you're working out, you want to get as close to 100 percent as possible.

Breathing properly is a basic, essential key to any exercise routine. Your body needs oxygen, and it's not going to come from anywhere else. Your body needs energy, and the fuel you put in your stomach is only part of it. This is the other part.

Breathe deeply through your nose. "Deeply" doesn't mean jerking your shoulders upward to draw a big breath. It means breathing from the *bottom* of your lungs, from the diaphragm. Expand your chest as far as you can. (As you "learn" to breathe, you're actually going to expand your rib cage and improve your posture.) While you're learning, you might even get a little light-headed—because you'll be high on oxygen.

There is an important rhythm to breathing while doing a routine. The best way to remember it is to *blow out on exertion*—in other words to exhale, strongly, during the hardest part of the movement. If you're doing bench presses, for example, blow out while you're raising the bar; inhale while bringing it back down. Practice the concept right now by doing some curling motions with your forearm. Force yourself to blow out while bringing your forearm up to your shoulder; inhale while lowering your arm. It might be just the opposite of your first inclination; but you'll feel the proper pattern, and get in tune with it, in just a couple of tries.

In the early days of your program, think about your breathing pattern constantly. Soon you'll be doing it right without thinking.

Remember, too, that proper breathing not only gets oxygen to your cells, it helps get wastes carried away. If you don't breathe efficiently, you're going to be much more sore the next day. That's why all those huffing and puffing aerobic dancers avoid post-workout pain.

BODY PARTS

Being fit gets you in touch with your body. Designing a workout program gets you in touch with your muscles in an almost clinical, analytical way. There are six major muscle groups to be worked, and every exercise is aimed at one or two of them. More advanced exercises are aimed at specific parts of one muscle. In the routines I've designed, beginners work on all six major groupings in each session. As you become more advanced, and the work becomes more intense, that number decreases. For example, in my own training I work on two body parts per session.

The major groupings are chest, triceps, legs, back, shoulders, biceps. There are subgroupings, of course, such as calves and stomach. The object of a good beginner's program is to train—in a plain, simple, fun fashion—the entire body in a symmetrical way.

Study. Ask questions. Resistance training, in all of its forms, has very specific goals for each movement. Know what it is that you are accomplishing, and you'll have more motivation to get it done.

REPS AND SETS

This is where you keep score. Except the goal isn't to "beat" the prescribed number of reps and sets. It's to do them exactly as programmed. As you progress, the program changes.

You'll see that the guts of each workout look incredibly simple: so many sets of a certain exercise, so many repetitions per set. But those numbers are very important. The number of repetitions in a set of a particular resistance exercise, in fact, determines what it is that you are doing to your body.

Here are the basic principles of reps—keeping in mind that more reps, of course, are done with less weight; and that larger muscles can handle, and need, more sets.

Is strength all you want? Do you want to bulk up? Then pure, unadulterated anaerobic exercise—quick, maximum bursts of effort—is the ticket. The power-lifters, the grunters for whom how many pounds they can hoist into the air is everything, look at eight reps as a *long* set.

Is definition and endurance your goal? You want to get your musculature "cut" or "ripped"? Then you're looking at basic sets of about 15 reps.

For me, 10 is a magic number. A set of 10 reps builds strength and builds muscle, but it also builds definition. In any basic program, think of sets made up of 10 reps each. Muscles that need more work get more sets.

Ten reps is a number *infinitely* more important than the number of pounds you are lifting. Gauge it this way, no matter what movement you are making: The eighth, ninth and 10th reps should be difficult. (To the point where an 11th might not be possible, or only with utmost effort.) When you are fitting that formula, the work you are doing is right for that muscle—whether the weight on the bar says 50 or 300. Ten is a magic number, and might be the most important thing to remember from this entire chapter.

Never sacrifice style for weight. If your biorhythms are down, or if maybe you haven't been able to get as much sleep as you should, remove some pounds from the bar if that's what it takes to get to 10. On the other hand, if you do 10 reps and put the bar down when you could be doing five more—then you should have added weight a long time ago.

Ten reps will break down muscle and stimulate growth of new, larger, stronger tissue. Remember to blow out on the toughest part of every movement, oxidizing the blood with each thrust of energy.

The number of sets is largely determined by the size of the muscle. The smaller the muscle, the quicker it will become over-trained. That's why a program might call for six sets of a shoulder exercise, and 12 or 15 sets for a leg exercise.

Don't forget that every single principle of reps and sets applies to manual resistance training—Dynabands and towels and broomsticks. The magic number is still 10. And if you're a couch potato, you'll actually be getting enough resistance to build muscle.

REST

Two different kinds of rest are vital to any workout program: rest between sets, and rest between workouts. Beginners need more of both.

Taking no more than 30 to 60 seconds between sets keeps you from losing the "pump"—from losing oxygen-rich blood flow to the muscles you are working. Beginners will need all 60 seconds as a target rest period. If you're far enough out of shape, you'll not only be sucking wind, you'll hit your anaerobic threshold. You might experience some nausea, dizziness, headache, a cold sweat. If you lose your cookies, you won't be the first.

Maybe not even the first of the day. It's very normal. It's your body saying: "Wait a minute!"

You have to start out by getting your mind in tune with the fact that this is, say, a 40-minute workout; that it's a lot more than just the first exercise. Then you have to push your body, but not kill it. Let me try to put all this in perspective by telling you what typically happens with personal training clients who come straight from 30 years at the office to their first day in a conditioning program. What I try to do—what all good personal trainers do—is try to work them to the max, short of hitting that wall. They come in all rambunctious. They're paying me by the hour. They want to get it on. But I fake them out a little, give them as much confidence as possible, keep them from feeling intimidated—but only give them *half* the workout. Next time, they get more.

Get the picture? You are the sculptor in every step of this conditioning process. You will constantly get in greater touch with your body. In the first workout or two, it might be more like your body slapping you in the face. You have to have patience with your body, listen to it, push it but don't insult it. You have to *wean* into fitness. You want to be back in the gym again and again for the rest of your life. Don't intimidate your body into refusing to bring you back.

I do "instinctive training." If I'm supposed to be doing five sets of one particular exercise, and if I lose "the pump" after four sets, I drop it. I move on. I've reached the plateau for that exercise. It takes years to be that in tune with your body. It's worth it in so many ways. Like when peer pressure or convenience tells you to pick up a double cheeseburger. A fit body tells you many things you can't hear just yet.

Rest between workouts is also crucial. A beginner will need 24 to 36 hours to recuperate. It takes me 12 hours—but again, it took me years to get to that point. Most beginners I put on a three-day-a-week program, two exercises per body part, two to three sets per exercise, 10 reps per set, 30 to 60 seconds between sets. That will build a foundation. There will be soreness in the first few rest days, but it will quickly diminish as you continue to work out.

SUPERSETS, TRI SETS, GIANT SETS

These exercises have a kind of Superman sound to them, but they are really just the opposite of power-lifting. They add aerobics and endurance conditioning to resistance training. They are very effective for athletes in endurance sports, who also want to add to their strength. I used supersetting, for example, to help condition a pro basketball player who was coming back from an Achilles tendon injury.

Supersets are nothing more than two different exercises, one set each, done back to back without rest. I use supersets myself for aerobic conditioning. And in the final weeks before a bodybuilding competition I use tri sets (three exercises back to back with no rest) and giant sets (four or more) to add tremendous definition to the musculature I have built in months of workouts.

The intensity in supersetting is immense, but there's no reason to be wary. The most effective supersetting is done on the *same* body part—chest, for example—in two different exercises. You'll be dissecting the muscle, exercising it in separate places, using its reserve energy and bringing it to maximum exhaustion. That's the key.

Any workout should aim to get in and out of the gym quickly—building muscle without overtraining, or getting stale, or getting bored. Neither you nor your muscle will get bored with supersets. In fact, you'll "confuse" the muscle and fake out its "memory"— the reason your body becomes immune to a single exercise routine if you follow it too long.

A superset shocks the body, throws it a curveball. Doing two different exercises back to back with *no rest* moves the intensity from second gear to fifth gear. You'll be cross-training, doing aerobics and anaerobics simultaneously.

You use less weight and, once again, the magic number of 10. When you complete one superset, you take the usual rest period (30 to 40 seconds, because you'll be conditioned before you do supersets). That's a fast pace, and you'll probably be sucking wind. Your cardiovascular endurance will thank you for it.

Bodybuilders aren't building muscle with supersets and lighter weights, they're sculpturing—which is why it's a pre-contest routine. As a combined endurance/strength workout, it's dynamite for a triathlete, a downhill skier, a tennis player or a basketball player.

Because of supersetting's aerobics component, it's also the perfect exercise for someone who wants resistance training but also wants to lose some weight. A moderate-carb protein-adequate, low-fat nutrition regimen and a gym regimen of supersets will make him or her one lean person.

SAFETY

Gyms can be dangerous places. So can cars. Defensive drivers who wear their seat belts shouldn't be afraid to drive to the grocery store. So it goes with gym training.

Some basic points:

• Make sure you are constantly bending your knees while doing any standing exercises. Your knees will act as a shock absorber. Otherwise your back will take the weight like throwing cement into a truck with no springs.

• Don't lock out on certain movements. For example, military shoulder presses, squats, leg presses.

• Wear a belt that's four inches wide. It'll also help protect your back. Anything wider than four inches will limit your range of motion.

• If you don't want calluses, wear a snug pair of gloves. If you wish, use a little chalk for a better grip.

• Wear loose clothing. You want good circulation and ventilation. Your arm can expand as much as an inch or inch and a half in the course of a workout, by the way.

• Wear sneakers or running shoes, with the laces well-tied. You want support and you don't want to trip.

• Wear gym socks to absorb sweat so you don't get bacterial infection.

• Always use a collar on a bar or adjustable dumbbell and fasten it tight to keep weights secure. That seems simple enough, but I've seen careless people splatter their face with a dumbbell.

• When you're walking around a gym don't lean against equipment unless you very consciously know exactly what the equipment is and what you are doing. Gym equipment has moveable parts. Some are chain-driven, for example. You could leave a finger in there if someone decided to lift while your hand was in the way.

• Keep a towel to wipe off your own sweat, or somebody else's, from a device or a bar you are about to grip or a bench you are about to lie on.

• Don't work beyond your comfort zone in hot and humid weather. "No pain no gain"—if you follow it out the window—is a fallacy. If something is painful while you're exercising, slow down or stop until the pain subsides. Overuse of muscles can cause damage or make you abandon your program.

DIARY

Whether it's a 49-cent spiral notebook or an executive logbook, this is one powerful tool. To my mind, it's absolutely essential for a successful program. You *are* going to make progress. But without a diary, you'll be at times like a ship passenger looking out at the ocean to see how far you've gone.

Use the diary to keep an accurate record of when you work out, what exercises you do, how many sets and reps, what poundage you use. Keep notes of what seems to be working and what doesn't. At the end of a session, if you think you're ready to make a change in a particular exercise next time, note it down so that you do. Write down questions you want to ask a trainer or instructor who isn't handy at the moment.

You might find it useful to combine a nutritional diary with your exercise diary. You should be keeping both. Some people find it easiest to put them in the same place; some find it more difficult.

Progress is all about goal-setting. After you've worked out a few months, and you hit a psychological down point (we all do), almost nothing will help you out as much as looking in your log. You'll see where you were. You'll remember why you're doing this. And you'll understand that, yes, you're getting there.

Real Bodybuilding

When you mention bodybuilding, people immediately think Arnold Schwartzenegger or the musclehead down at the gym, but the truth is we all need to be bodybuilders. Whether someone wants to put on muscle, take off weight, or just get healthy after an illness, we all need to build our bodies. Our bodies were made to move, they were made to actively engage in life. When the body isn't active it atrophies and breaks down. So, by all means I want you to become a body builder! Build it into the best you it can be! Don't be in competition with anyone. In this contest it's you against you.

The wise are the winners when it comes to beginning a workout program. Start slow and stay basic in the beginning.

Below is a sample workout for any beginner, even if you've never picked up a weight. Following this routine will get you out of the starting blocks and into the race, and trust me, once you're in the race you'll never again want to be on the sidelines!

Remember, this isn't about lifting tons of weight, it's about reps, and the magic number is 10! Don't start too big and injure yourself. Keep your target at ten reps.

All of my beginner's programs are designed for three days a week, Monday-Wednesday-Friday or Tuesday-Thursday-Saturday. The two off days are needed for a proper cycle of rest. This program will produce results for anyone. It's basic no nonsense exercises that are tried and true. Arnold used them, I use them, and you can too!

Chest:	Exercise:
A: 2 sets of 10 reps	A: Inclined bench press with barbell
B: 2 sets of 10 reps	B: Flat dumbbell flye

For the bench press, use a 45 degree incline. Lie back and hold a weighted barbell at arms' length. You will want your grip slightly beyond shoulder length. Lower the bar lightly touching it against the upper chest, then press back upward until arms are straight. Remember to blow out on exertion, going up.

For the flye, lie on back on flat bench holding a dumbbell in each hand above the chest with palms-in grip. Slowly lower the weights out and down until the arms are parallel to the floor. You will want to maintain a slight bend in the arms to avoid hurting arms or shoulders. When the chest is fully stretched, change direction and raise weights back up, tightening your chest muscles.

Back:	Exercise:
A: 2 sets of 10 reps	A: Wide-grip barbell bend-over rows
B: 2 sets of 10 reps	B: Lat machine pulldown behind neck

For the bent-over rows, stand on the floor or on a raised platform to get more of a stretch. Bend forward, keeping knees slightly bent. Grasp weighted barbell with a wide overhand grip and lift bar slightly while your back is parallel to the floor. Keeping back flat, exhale and bend arms to lift the bar until it is near the stomach. Inhale as you lower bar to starting position without letting the weight touch the floor. That's one rep.

For the pulldowns, sit at a lat pulldown machine gripping the long bar with a wide open-handed grip. Place your thighs under the pads to hold the body down as you pull. Begin with arms straight over your head. Pull down by bending the elbows and squeezing the lat, stopping when the bar touches the back of the neck. Stretch the arms back out and repeat.

Triceps:	Exercise:
A: 2 sets of 10 reps	A: Dumbbell kickbacks
B: 2 sets of 10 reps	B: Triceps dips

For the kickbacks, grasp a dumbbell you can handle easily with one arm. Assume a bent-over position on a bench or stool or chair. Place one foot 12 inches in front of the other, with your upper body parallel to the floor. Hold the dumbbell with an over-hand grip, taking care to keep your upper body and elbow in line, with your forearm hanging straight down. That's the position.

The movement: While keeping your body still and upper arm tucked into your side, exhale and extend the arm (the only part of the arm that's moving is from elbow to wrist) to the rear until the arm is straight back. Inhale and return the dumbbell to the bottom positions. After doing 10 reps, switch arms. The arm will work the entire triceps.

For the dips, place two benches parallel and three to four feet apart. Support yourself on both benches--legs straight out and feet on one bench, hands behind hips on the other bench. Keeping the upper body erect, bend the elbows and lower your buttocks down near the floor. Use triceps to push back to straight-arm position. Inhale moving down; exhale moving up. Squeeze triceps at the top. For added resistance you can place a weighted dumbbell or weight on your thighs. You can also do this exercise at home using chairs or a bed.

Biceps:	Exercise:
A: 2 sets of 10 reps	A: Standing barbell curls (medium grip)
B: 2 sets of 10 reps	B: Alternate dumbbell curls, seated

For the barbell curls, Stand with feet at shoulder width, gripping the bar at thigh level-- with elbows nearly straight, palms facing upward and hands just outside the hips. Keeping the back straight, exhale and curl bar up to chest by bending elbows. Stop when biceps become fully tight, and do not let them relax by resting the bar against your chest. Lower bar while inhaling. This classic exercise is excellent for building big biceps.

For the alternate dumbbell curls, sit upright on a bench or chair holding a dumbbell in each hand with a palms-in grip. Keeping the right hand immobile, twist the left hand so palm faces you and lift the dumbbell by bending the elbow. Squeeze at the top so you are flexing the muscle. Repeat with opposite arm and continue to alternate.

Shoulders:	Exercise:
A: 2 sets of 10 reps	A: Seated military shoulder press
B: 2 sets of 10 reps	B: Dumbbell side lateral

For the press, sit on a flat bench with barbell resting on shoulders and grip the bar beyond shoulder width with palms facing forward. Keep back straight and feet planted firmly on the floor. Exhale as you press the bar to arms' length in a controlled manner. Inhale and slowly return the bar to starting position.

For the lateral, stand with legs spread wide, knees slightly bent and back upright. Hold a dumbbell in each hand with palms facing the body. Breathing through your nose, inhale as you slowly raise dumbbells up and out to the sides, stopping when arms are at ear height. Hold for a count of three seconds, then slowly lower weights back to starting position. Keep thumbs pointed upward at all times. Never lift above your head in this exercise.

Legs:	Exercise:
A: 2 sets of 10 reps	A: Leg extensions
B: 2 sets of 10 reps	B: Leg curls

Extensions will build the outer front thigh, the quadriceps. Sit at a leg extension machine with your insteps behind the roller pads and your hands gripping the handles at the side of machine. Slowly straighten legs to life the weights, keeping toes pointed up. Stop when knees are locked and quadriceps are flexed. Pause and lower, under control, to starting position without letting the weights come to rest.

This exercise increases overall knee strength, boosts vertical jump and helps running speed. Be sure to adjust the leg extension seat so the back of the knee is snug against the front edge of seat. The bottom pad should be just above the ankle area but below the shin. Keeping your toes standing at attention makes sure that you work the entire quadriceps. Use a fluid, slow motion.

For the second exercise, lie on a leg hamstring curl machine with your heels beneath the roller pad and your chest flat on the bench pad, holding handles for support. Exhale and bend knees to lift pad as far as possible. Hold the flexed position momentarily before inhaling and lowering to starting position. The kneecap should be just off the pad, or you'll hurt your knees. Keeping the heel tucked in isolates the muscle you're working. Make sure that it's a fully controlled fluid motion.

Stomach:	Nielsen's tri set:
2 Giant sets, all to failure	A: Leg raises on stand
	B: Crunches (legs on bench)
	C: Sit-ups on board

Unlike all the other muscles, the stomach area should be worked to failure instead of counting reps and resting between sets. As soon as you reach failure on one exercise, you move on to the next.

First, do leg raises on a legstand and work the stomach from the belly button down, attacking that little pouch area that a lot of people want to tone up. Because they work the lower abs best, knee-tuck leg raises should be done first in your routine. Position yourself on a standing abdominal chair, supporting body weight on the forearms and hanging the straightened legs downward. Keeping your knees nearly straight, exhale and bend at the hips, lifting the legs out and up in front of you until they are parallel to the floor. Pause and inhale while returning to starting position. Immediately repeat, using a slow motion to work the abs better and ease strain off the lower back.

Next do crunches with your legs on a bench and your back firmly on the floor so your body lies in three nearly straight lines--torso on the floor, hips to knees straight upward, knees to feet on the bench and parallel to the floor. Position your buttocks very near the bench (or the bed or couch; this is an exercise you can easily do at home). Make relaxed fists and cross your hands on your chest to centralize your weight.

Your arms weigh at least three to five pounds, and you don't want to put them behind your head as in a traditional sit-up. To start, push your neck forward, then, from the middle of your back to the shoulders, raise your upper torso three to four inches and *squeeze* (simultaneously blowing out). That's the crunch.

For the sit-ups, never use a board slanted more than 45 degrees. This exercise works the entire stomach, but again focuses from the belly button upward. Again, centralize your weight by crossing your fists over your chest. Sitting on a slanted board, go down just halfway, inhaling. Blow out as you come up fully and extend your neck so you're actually squeezing stomach muscles. As you blow out, you constrict stomach muscles and put tension from you own weight on your abdominals. Do this to failure--till you get that burn in your stomach.

Calves:	Exercise:
3 sets of 10	Seated calf raises

Sit on a calf raising machine with your knees under the pads and the balls of your feet on the front platform. Lift weights by raising the toes. Unlock the holding bar. Begin with heels lowered so that the calves are stretched. Exhale and lift the weight by flexing the calves and lifting heels as high as possible. Squeeze momentarily, then lower to stretch position while inhaling. Do three sets: first with feet straight, second with toes and feet facing inward, third with feet facing outward. This develops the full calf muscle.

These exercises are simple, effective and proven to produce results every time if done properly and consistently.

RECOMMENDED LINKS

I urge you to continue in your quest for healing and wholeness by referring to the links below.

Principles of Hope website: http://principlesofhope.com/

Principles of Hope facebook page:
https://www.facebook.com/pages/Principles-of-Hope/266504550054343

Peter's Principles website: http://www.petersprinciples.com/

LifeCare Christian Center website: www.LifeCareChristianCenter.org

For prayer, donations, partnership, support or to order materials or ask questions,

contact our call center at

1-800-HOPE-361

CHILD ABUSE IN THE UNITED STATES: How Bad Is It?

Every Day, Four Children Die from Abuse in the United States. Every year, 3 million cases of child abuse, involving 6 million children, are reported. And as many as a half million more cases of abuse may go unreported each year.

THIS IS A HIDDEN EPIDEMIC! Our society should be up in arms over and fighting each and every day. Where is the outrage??? Who is championing the cause? If nothing changes to rescue these poor, helpless children, another 1,500 children will die from abuse this year. It's time to speak up—and stand up—for these children. **We cannot remain silent!**

Just imagine, if we save 20 percent of the 500,000 children whose abuse goes unreported every year, we will have saved a number equal to the entire population of a major city such as Ann Arbor, Michigan; Allentown, Pennsylvania; Abilene, Texas; or Berkley, California. **That's 100,000 children!**

Also consider that there are hundreds of agencies that help children *after* they have been abused and rescued from hostile environments. However, there are very few organizations educating the public on how to spot and report abuse.

Our Child Abuse Prevention Kit fills this void.

This kit teaches you about the seriousness of the child abuse epidemic, shows you signs to look for so you can spot an abuse case, and informs you on how and where to report it, no matter where you live.

Our Child Abuse Prevention Kit helps you make that call to help save abused children.

The little bit of discomfort or inconvenience you may feel while making the call to report child abuse is nothing compared with the suffering that child continues to feel if you don't make that call. We urge everyone to be on the lookout and make that rescuing call.

Learn how to stop child abuse by visiting 2saveachild.org

When you make a tax deductible donation, you are giving an abused child new hope and a better life. Please donate now.

CAP Kit, Inc.
23136 Hughes
Suite A
Hazel Park, MI 48030

REFERENCES

Beecher, Henry Ward.
http://thinkexist.com/quotation/what_a_mother_sings_to_the_cradle_goes_all_the/782
9.html.

Bounds, E.M. *The Complete Works of E.M. Bounds*. Wilder Publications: 2009.

"Dear Dad in the Recliner." November 13, 2012.
http://4littlefergusons.wordpress.com/2012/11/13/dear-dad-in-the-recliner/.

"Dear Mom On the iPhone." November 14, 2012.
http://4littlefergusons.wordpress.com/?s=dear+mom+on+the+iphone&submit=Search.

Denos, Matthew. http://www.beliefnet.com/Health/Why-Eating-Right-and-Exercising-
Glorifies-God.aspx.

Dulyan, Aram. December 9, 2003. Verrazano Narrows Bridge, New York, NY, USA.
http://zh.wikipedia.org/zh-hans/File:Verrazano-Bridge-Dawn.jpg.

Finn, Charles C. "Please Hear What I'm Not Saying" adapted.
http://www.poetrybycharlescfinn.com/pleasehear.html. September, 1966.

Flanigan, Beverly. *Forgiving the Unforgivable: Overcoming the Bitter Legacy of Intimate
Wounds*. Wiley: 1994.

Footprints in the Sand. http://www.poem4today.com/footprints-poem.html.

Footprints variation. http://www.pinterest.com/pin/245727723390866775/.

Gurnall, William. *The Christian in Complete Armour*. Hendrickson Publishing: Reprint
edition, 2010.

Ingram, Chip. *Living on the Edge Ministries*.

King, Jr., Dr. Martin Luther.
http://www.brainyquote.com/quotes/quotes/m/martinluth103425.html. Nietzsche,
Friedrich. http://www.brainyquote.com/quotes/quotes/f/friedrichn105845.html.

Lockwood Huie, Jonathan. http://www.jonathanlockwoodhuie.com/quote/today-choose-
higher-road-path-121/.

Luebering, Carol. "Finding a way to forgive." *CareNotes* #20653.
    http://www.onecaringplace.com/product.asp?pn=20653.

MPAA rating system has become more lenient, How and why.
    http://www.examiner.com/article/how-and-why-mpaa-rating-system-has-become-more-lenient.

Nielsen, Peter N. *Will of Iron*. Royal Oak, MI: Momentum Books LLC, 2005: 61-64, 107-120, 149-165, 170-174.

Ramsey, Dave.
    http://www.daveramsey.com/index.cfm?event=askdave/&intContentItemId=120533.

Reagan, Ronald. http://www.brainyquote.com/quotes/quotes/r/ronaldreag183750.html.

Sledge, Tim. *Making Peace With Your Past*. Nashville: LifeWay Press, 1992.

Smedes, Lewis B. http://www.brainyquote.com/quotes/quotes/l/lewisbsme132886.html.

Spurgeon, Charles. http://christian-quotes.ochristian.com/christian-quotes_ochristian.cgi?query=trust&action=search.

Stanley, Charles. http://www.christianindex.org/2431.article.

Stanley, Charles. http://www.intouch.org/Content/27938/LP110515.pdf.

Swindoll, Chuck. http://www.brainyquote.com/quotes/quotes/c/charlesrs155778.html.

Thurman, Dr. Chris. *The Lies We Believe*. Thomas Nelson (reprint ed.): 2003.

Wiersbe, Warren. http://www.searchquotes.com/quotes/author/Warren_Wiersbe/.

Yancey, Philip. "The Unnatural Act". *Christianity Today*. April 8, 1991.

Made in the USA
Middletown, DE
18 May 2016